*ti***O** *Techniques in Orthopaedics*

Editorial Board

Lester Borden, M.D.
Cleveland, Ohio

Kenneth E. DeHaven, M.D.
Rochester, New York

Lawrence D. Dorr, M.D.
Downey, California

David S. Hungerford, M.D.
Baltimore, Maryland

William Grana, M.D.
Oklahoma City, Oklahoma

Douglas W. Jackson, M.D.
Long Beach, California

James Kellam, M.D.
Toronto, Ontario, Canada

John B. McGinty, M.D.
Newton Lower Falls, Massachusetts

Chitranjan S. Ranawat, M.D.
New York, New York

David Seligson, M.D.
Louisville, Kentucky

Phillip G. Spiegel, M.D.
Tampa, Florida

Richard B. Welch, M.D.
San Francisco, California

Robert A. Winquist, M.D.
Seattle, Washington

Techniques in Orthopaedics

Topics in Orthopaedic Trauma

Phillip G. Spiegel, M.D.

Professor and Chairman
Department of Orthopaedic Surgery
University of South Florida
College of Medicine
Tampa, Florida

University Park Press • Baltimore

University Park Press
International Publishers in Medicine and Human Services
300 North Charles Street
Baltimore, Maryland 21201

Copyright © 1984 by University Park Press

This book is protected by copyright. All rights, including that of translation into other languages are reserved. No part of this book may be reproduced, stored in a retrieval system, or transmitted in any form or by any means, electronic, mechanical, photocopying, recording, or otherwise, without the prior written permission of the publisher.

Sponsoring Editor: Larry W. Carter
Production Manager: Berta Steiner
Cover and text design: Caliber Design Planning, Inc.

Typeset by Kingsport Press
Manufactured in the United States of America by Halliday Lithograph

0–8391–1977–1

Contents

Preface   *vii*

Contributors   *ix*

1   **Acute Management of Fractures and Dislocations of the Cervical Spine: A Correlative Approach**   **1**

   William A. Teipner, Jeffrey W. Mast, and Neal H. Shonnard

2   **Supracondylar and Intercondylar Fractures of the Adult Humerus**   **21**

   Marshall Horowitz

3   **Small ASIF External Fixator for Fractures of the Wrist and Further Applications**   **35**

   Roland P. Jakob

4   **Stabilizing Hand Fractures with Tension Bands**   **57**

   Robert Belsole

5   **Multiple Trauma and Pelvic Bleeding: Diagnosis and Treatment**   **69**

   R. Y. McMurtry

6   **Ender Nailing of Intertrochanteric Fractures of the Femur**   **77**

   James P. Waddell

Contents

7 Ipsilateral Hip and Femur Fractures: Methods of Treatment 85

Frank F. Cook, James C. Binski, and Marshall Horowitz

8 Preoperative Planning of Corrective Surgery for Posttraumatic Deformities in the Adult 99

Jeffrey W. Mast, William A. Teipner, and Aaron A. Hofmann

9 Femur Fractures with Simultaneous Knee Ligament Injuries 117

Arthur K. Walling, Houshang Seradge, and Phillip G. Spiegel

10 Dislocation of the Knee in the Competitive Athlete 125

J. R. Steadman and James B. Montgomery

11 Fixation of Tibial Shaft Fractures with Flexible Intramedullary Nails 135

Arsen M. Pankovich

12 External Fixation of Fibular Fractures 145

Richard A. Fischer and David Seligson

13 Triplane Fractures of the Distal Tibial Epiphysis 153

Phillip G. Spiegel, Jeffrey W. Mast, Daniel R. Cooperman, and Gerald S. Laros

14 Open Reduction and Internal Fixation of Calcaneus Fractures 173

Emile Letournel

15 Internal Fixation of Nonunions After Previously Unsuccessful Electromagnetic Stimulation 193

Howard Rosen

Index 209

Preface

The primary purpose of this volume is to assist the practicing orthopaedic surgeon in the up-to-date management of specific trauma problems. The topics were chosen for their timeliness, usefulness, and relevancy. The authors personal experience, methods and techniques are highlighted in each article. Glimpses of future directions in the care of acute and chronic trauma problems are also included to be used as alternative suggestions to present day fracture management.

The volume should be read as one would read a collection of short stories: each article a self-contained unit of knowledge, to be read again when that specific problem presents itself. Hopefully, a satisfied patient will be the happy ending to each "story" told.

The editor would like to express his thanks to the authors for their unique contributions to the orthopaedic literature and to Ms. Deborah Smelt for her invaluable editorial assistance.

PGS

Contributors

Robert Belsole, M.D.
Associate Professor
Department of Orthopaedic Surgery
University of South Florida College of Medicine
12901 N. 30th Street, Box 36
Tampa, Florida 33612

James C. Binski, M.D.
Chief, Division of Reconstructive Surgery
Department of Orthopaedic Surgery
University Hospital
580 W. 8th Street
Jacksonville, Florida 32209

Frank F. Cook, M.D.
Department of Orthopaedic Surgery
University Hospital
580 W. 8th Street
Jacksonville, Florida 32209

Daniel R. Cooperman, M.D.
Assistant Professor of Surgery (Orthopaedics)
University of Chicago
The Pritzker School of Medicine
950 E. 59th Street
Chicago, Illinois 60637

Richard A. Fischer, M.D.
Department of Orthopaedics and Rehabilitation
University of Vermont
Burlington, Vermont 05405

Aaron A. Hofmann, M.D.
Assistant Professor of Orthopaedics
Division of Orthopaedic Surgery
University of Utah Medical Center
50 North Medical Drive
Salt Lake City, Utah 84132

Marshall Horowitz, M.D.
Chairman
Department of Orthopaedic Surgery
University Hospital
580 West 8th Street
Jacksonville, Florida 32209

Roland P. Jakob, M.D.
Universitatsklinik fur orthopaedische Chirurgie
Inselspital
CH-3010 Bern, Switzerland

Gerald S. Laros, M.D.
Professor of Surgery (Orthopaedics)
University of Chicago
The Pritzker School of Medicine
950 E. 59th Street
Chicago, Illinois 60637

Emile Letournel
Professor Agrege of Orthopaedics
and Traumatology
10 Rue Angelique
Verien n. Neuilly S.
Seine 92200, France

Jeffrey W. Mast, M.D.
Associate Clinical Professor of Surgery
University of Nevada Medical School
555 N. Arlington Avenue
Reno, Nevada 89520

R. Y. McMurtry, M.D.
Assistant Professor of Orthopaedic Surgery
University of Toronto
2075 Bayview Avenue
Room G 394
Toronto, Ontario M4N 3M5, Canada

James B. Montgomery, M.D.
Assistant Professor
Department of Surgery
Division of Orthopaedic Surgery
University of Texas
Health Science Center
5323 Harry Hines Blvd.
Dallas, Texas 75235

Arsen Pankovich, M.D.
Professor of Orthopaedic Surgery
Kings County Hospital
C-11
451 Clarkson Avenue
Brooklyn, New York 11203

Howard Rosen, M.D.
Clinical Professor of Orthopaedic Surgery
Mt. Sinai School of Medicine
1 Gustad L. Levy Place
New York, New York 10029

David Seligson, M.D.
Kosair Professor and Chairman
Division of Orthopaedics

University of Louisville School of Medicine
550 S. Jackson Street
Louisville, Kentucky 40292

Houshang Seradge, M.D.
Clinical Assistant Professor of Orthopaedic Surgery
University of Oklahoma
Health Sciences Center
1044 S.W. 44th Street
Oklahoma City, Oklahoma 73109

Neal H. Shonnard
University of Nevada Medical School
555 North Arlington Avenue
Reno, Nevada 89520

Phillip G. Spiegel, M.D.
Professor and Chairman
Department of Orthopaedic Surgery
University of South Florida
College of Medicine
Tampa, Florida 33612

J. R. Steadman, M.D.
Assistant Clinical Professor of Orthopaedic Surgery
University of Nevada-Reno
Reno, Nevada 89520

William A. Teipner, M.D.
Associate Clinical Professor of Surgery
University of Nevada Medical School
555 North Arlington Avenue
Reno, Nevada 89520

Arthur Walling
Assistant Professor
Department of Orthopaedic Surgery
College of Medicine
University of South Florida
12901 N. 30th Street, Box 36
Tampa, Florida 33612

James P. Waddell, M.D.
Chief of Orthopaedics
St. Michael's Hospital
38 Shuter Street, Suite 507
Toronto, Ontario M5B 1A6, Canada

tiO *Techniques in Orthopaedics*

Acute Management of Fractures and Dislocations of the Cervical Spine: A Correlative Approach

1

William A. Teipner
Jeffrey W. Mast
Neal H. Shonnard

The treatment of fractures and dislocation of the cervical spine should relate to the more important neurologic deficit, whether it be a specific cord syndrome, a specific root involvement, or both. This factor takes precedence over the mechanism of injury and the column involvement in the surgical management of these patients.

When no neurologic deficit exists, the goal is to provide stabilization by the simplest approach, thereby allowing early mobilization of the patient and preventing late deformity and/or a neurologic deficit (Figures 1–1A,B).

Our observations are based on the experience of members of the Reno Orthopaedic Clinic with 134 cases treated from 1970 to 1982 (Table 1–1). We strongly believe in a protocol that utilizes a team approach, with the basic members being an orthopaedist, a neurosurgeon, and a rehabilitation specialist (see acknowledgment). Other specialists are consulted as needed to handle the many other problems encountered, particularly cardiorespiratory and genitourinary complications. A common philosophy must exist, particularly between the orthopedist and the neurosurgeon. There is no place for laminectomy alone as an isolated neurosurgical procedures except in rare circumstances associated with a penetrating injury (5,31,33).

Neurological Evaluation

Initial neurological evaluation of the patient is paramount when making a decision about the appropriate management of the injury. We are indebted to Schneider for his succinct classification of specific spinal cord syndromes (26–28). These syndromes relate to the specific injury in incomplete lesions of the spinal cord. The area of injury to the spinal cord is classified as to whether the damage is anterior, central, lateral, or posterior. With complete transection

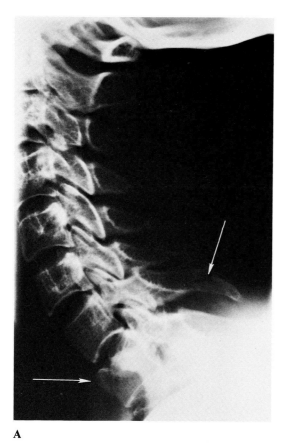 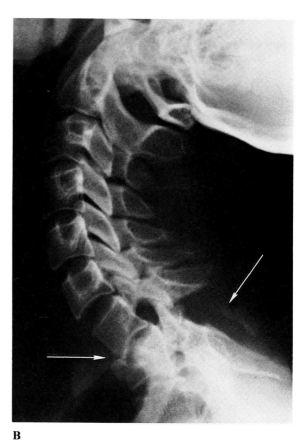

Figure 1–1 Posterior ligamentous disruption and compression fracture (*arrows*) with no neurologic deficit in a 24-year-old female) involved in a motor vehicle accident (MVA). **A** Injury x-ray. **B** Increasing pain and C8 nerve root involvement with late instability (*arrows*).

of the spinal cord, whether it be physiological or anatomic, our concern rests with preservation of as much nerve root function as possible.

The anterior cord syndrome may result from direct compression of the anterior spinal cord by a herniated disc or fracture-dislocation. Consequently, this syndrome is secondary to involvement of the spinothalamic and corticospinal tracts. It is associated with varying degrees of motor paralysis and loss of pain and temperature sensation below the level of the injury. Posterior column function is generally not affected in that the sensations of vibration, motion, and proprioception usually remain intact.

The central cord syndrome results from hemorrhage, edema, and/or necrosis of the central gray matter of the spinal cord. A hemorrhagic and edematous process may extend to adjacent white matter. This syndrome is secondary to involvement of anterior horn motor neurons and the more central portion of the corticospinal tracts. There is also a variable sensory loss, but bowel and bladder functions may be spared because of the more peripherally placed sacral pathways in the lateral columns of the spinal cord (*16*). The clinical features of this syndrome are characterized by a disproportionately greater weakness in the upper extremities compared to the lower extremities. This is due to compromise of the more centrally placed upper extremity motor fibers in the corticospinal tracts.

Cervical Spine Fractures

Table 1–1. Fractures/Dislocations of the Cervical Spine in 134 Patients

Sex	No.	Meanage (yr)	Mechanism of injury	
M	110	31.4 (7–74)	MVA	89
F	24	34.6 (13–77)	Fall	17
			Diving	13
Neurologic evaluation			Athletics	15
No deficit	52 (39%)		**Type of neurological deficit**	
Deficit	82 (61%)			
			Complete cord	21
Anatomic distribution of injuries			Central cord	10
			Anterior cord	10
C1	5 (3%)		Posterior cord	0
C1–C2 ligaments	2 (1%)		Brown-Sequard	10
Odontoid	22 (16%)		Nerve root	28
Type I	3		Transient findings	3
Type II	17			
Type III	2		**Type and frequency of mid/lower cervical spine injuries**	
Hangman's	13 (10%)			
Mid/lower cervical spine	95 (70%)			
			Unifacet	27 (28%)
Definitive treatment			Bifacet	13 (14%)
			Teardrop	28 (29%)
Closed	54 (40%)		Ligament	10 (11%)
Surgery (fusion)	80 (60%)		Ligament + compression fracture	12 (13%)
Anterior	16 (20%)			
Posterior	64 (80%)		Lateral mass	3 (3%)
Halo	90 (67%)		Disc rupture	2 (2%)
Brace	41 (30%)			

Deaths occurred in 7 (5%) of the patients, all of whom had cord syndromes: 5 patients with a complete cord syndrome and 2 with a central cord syndrome.

The lateral, or more commonly called Brown-Sequard, syndrome is seen after disproportionate damage occurs to one side of the cord. The ipsilateral corticospinal and spinothalamic tracts are involved, and the syndrome manifests as a greater motor loss on the ipsilateral side of the body and a contralateral loss of pain and temperature sensation below the level of the injury.

The posterior cord syndrome is rare and shows loss of the posterior column functions of proprioception and vibratory sense below the level of the cord injury. We had none in our series. These syndromes provide broad outlines in incomplete lesions and at times overlap.

Of next importance is the presence or absence of nerve root function at the level of the injury. This is important whether it be the isolated neurologic problem or associated with a complete or incomplete cord deficit. Sensory patterns are well known, as described in anatomy texts, with shoulder sensation intact at C4, upper arm and forearm at C5, thumb and index at C6, middle finger at C7, fourth and fifth digits at C8, and inner arm sensation at T1.

The important motor contributions to the upper extremity are: C4—trapezius and sternocleidomastoid; C5—deltoid and biceps; C6—radial wrist extensors; C7—triceps, finger extensors, and wrist flexors; C8—finger flexors and intrinsics; and T1—intrinsics (19).

Fracture Patterns

There are several common fracture types which can be easily identified (Figure 1–2). In the upper cervical spine, we identify the injuries as follows:

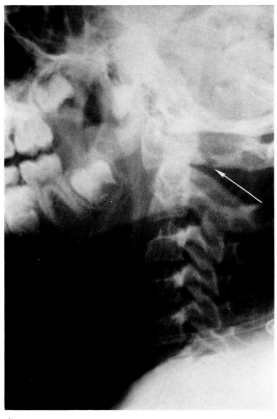 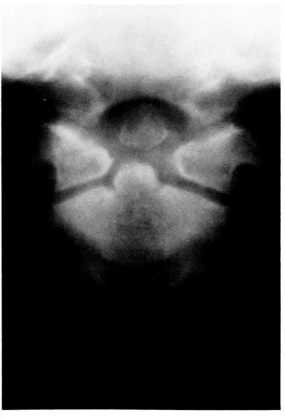

A B

Figure 1-2 Collage of fracture patterns. **A** Ring fracture of C1, called a Jefferson fracture (*arrow*). **B** Ostodontoidium, tomogram. **C** Fracture pars interarticular C2 (Hangman's fracture) with a fracture of the anteroinferior body of C2 (*arrows*). **D** Unilateral facet dislocation. **E** Tomogram of the patient in Figure 1-2D: uninvolved side (*arrow*). **F** Tomogram of the patient in Figure 1-2D: dislocated side (*arrow*).

1. *C1 ring fractures* (*20*)—most commonly consisting of a fracture of the posterior neural arch of C1, called a Jefferson fracture (Figure 1-2A).
2. *Odontoid fractures*—commonly classified into three basic types (*1*):
    Type I—a fracture through the odontoid in its mid or upper portion, which is frequently confused with the os odontoidium (Figure 1-2B), a more commonly encountered problem (*8,9*).
    Type II—a fracture at the base of the odontoid (Figure 1-3A, below).
    Type III—a fracture which extends into the body of C2.

We have also chosen to identify a fourth injury in this location which is a pure ligamentous subluxation of C1 on C2 (Table 1-1).

3. *Bilateral fracture of the pars interarticularis at C2* (*9*)—at times associated with a compression or avulsion fracture of the anterior body of C2 or C3, "traumatic spondylolisthesis" (*13*), or "Hangman's" fracture (*30*) (Figure 1-2C).

We identify the common fracture patterns seen in the mid and lower cervical spine as follows:

Cervical Spine Fractures

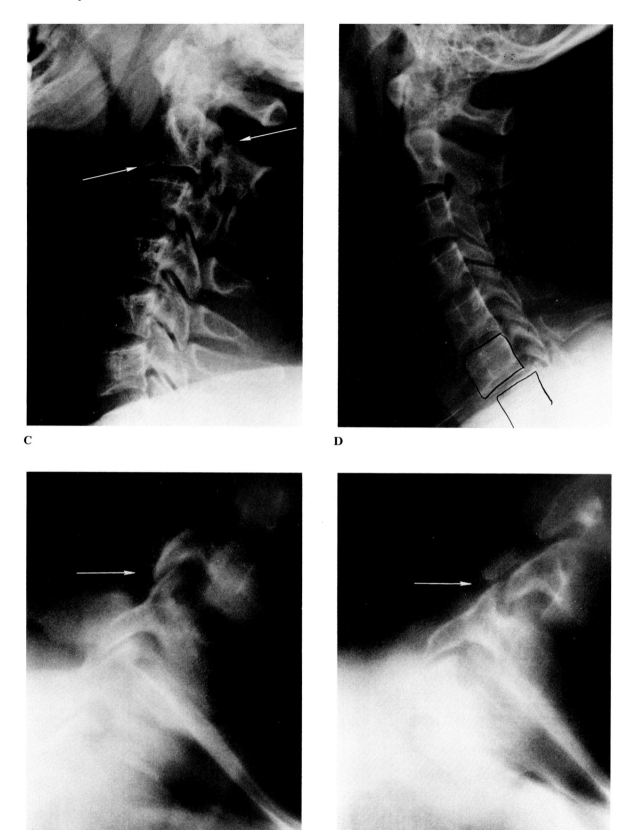

C

D

E

F

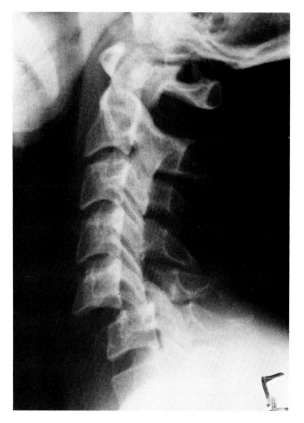

G

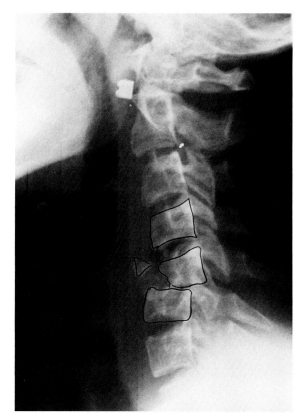

H

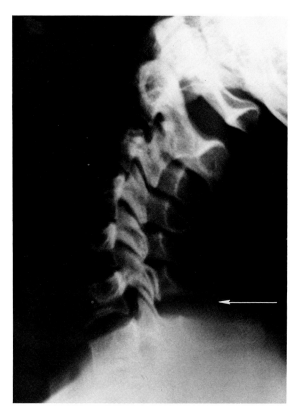

I

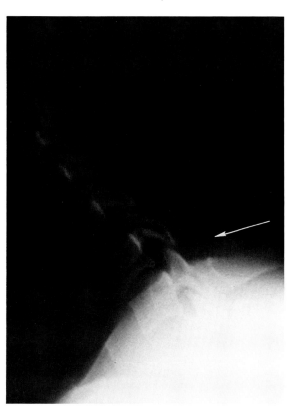

J

Cervical Spine Fractures

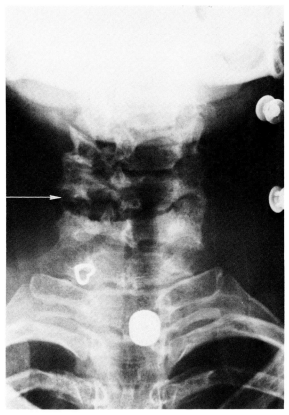 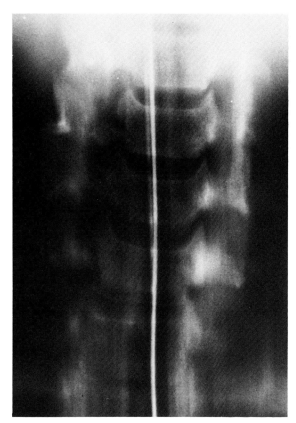

K L

Figure 1–2 (cont.) G Bilateral facet dislocation. **H** Flexion teardrop fracture dislocation/burst fracture. **I** Pure ligamentous disruption (extension) (*arrow*). **J** Pure ligamentous disruption (flexion) (*arrow*). **K** Lateral mass fracture (*arrow*). **L** Tomogram of the patient in Figure 1–2K.

1. *Unilateral facet fracture and/or dislocation.* This injury is frequently associated with a specific nerve root involvement; in our series it was seen in 16 of 27 cases (60%) (Figures 1–2D–F).
2. *Bilateral facet dislocation and/or fracture.* This injury has a high incidence of spinal cord injury (*32*); in our series it was seen in 10 of 13 cases (77%) (Figure 1–2G).
3. *Flexion teardrop fracture dislocation/burst fracture.* This frequently exhibits a triangular fragment broken off the anteroinferior portion of the involved body (*17,23,29*). The fracture may result from pure axial loading (*35*) or axial loading with flexion. This injury is associated with a very high incidence of spinal cord involvement (*25,26*); in our series it was seen in 23 of 28 cases (82%) (Figure 1–2H).
4. *Posterior ligamentous disruption.* This injury has a high propensity for late instability, and the instability at times goes unrecognized without appropriate flexion and extension x-ray views (Figures 1–2I,J).
5. *Posterior ligamentous disruption associated with a compression fracture at the level of injury* (Figure 1–1A). Again, this injury has a high propensity for late instability (Figure 1–1B).
6. *Lateral mass fracture.* In our experience this can be quite unpredictable as to the neurologic deficit (Figures 1–2K,L).

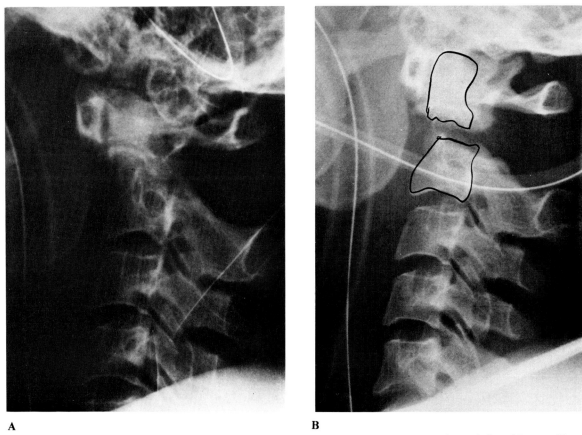

Figure 1–3 Unstable odontoid type II fracture with quadriparesis in a 39-year-old male involved in an MVA. **A** Odontoid fracture, type II. **B** Gardner-Wells traction.

Initial Treatment

After the history and physical examination are completed, and particularly after the neurologic evaluation, minimal scout films are ordered, the most important being a lateral x-ray that shows the anatomy down to and including C7 and T1. At times this requires the use of a special swimmer's view (*14*). With significant injuries skeletal traction is applied; currently our method of choice uses the Gardner-Wells tongs. At this point, more sophisticated studies can be done, including plain films, tomograms, a computed tomography (CT) scan, and occasionally a myelogram. A Stryker frame or a standard bed with some type of flotation mattress is utilized.

Decision-Making and Method of Stabilization in Various Fracture Types

Upper Cervical Spine

With fractures of the upper cervical spine where surgery is indicated, we have used exclusively a posterior surgical approach. The C1 (Jefferson) fracture (Figure 1–2A) can be treated with a closed method (*15*). The common posterior ring fracture is stable and can be managed with a Somi brace during

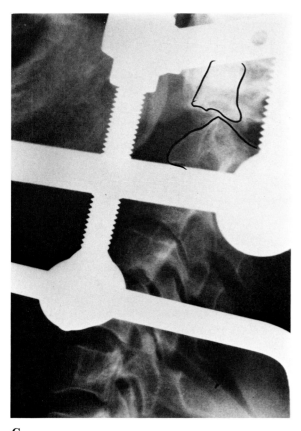 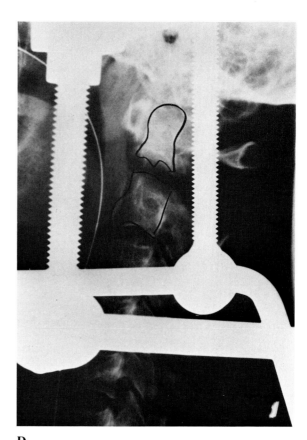

C D

Figure 1–3 (cont.) C Halo vest, unreduced fracture. D Halo vest, adjustment of reduction.

the day and a Philadelphia collar at night. Occasionally a halo vest is used for displaced unstable C1 ring fractures (39).

The odontoid fracture presents a different problem. The type I injury is rare and can be treated in a closed fashion (1,17), although the more commonly seen os odontoidium is frequently unstable (10) and requires posterior C1–C2 fusion (9,10) (Figure 1–2B).

The type II injury, occurring at the base of the odontoid when there is no significant displacement, has been managed in our hands and by others with a halo vest and a high rate of union (7,22,24). There were no nonunions of this specific injury if it was recognized early and treated promptly. On the other hand, if there is significant displacement present, we prefer C1–C2 posterior fusion (24) combined with a halo vest as the preferred method of postoperative immobilization (5,6). In these extremely unstable odontoid type II fractures, a preliminary halo vest is applied, obtaining as accurate a closed reduction as possible; this is followed by open posterior stabilization with fusion from C1 to C2 (Figure 1–3A–E). A flexion injury with anterior displacement of the odontoid is considerably easier to manage than an extension injury because of the ease of reduction and maintenance of the reduction of the former.

There are many acceptable techniques for wiring the posterior neural arch of C1 to C2 for an odontoid injury (2,12,24). Our preference, after exposure and decortication of the posterior neural arch of C1 and C2 with an air drill, involves the use of an 18-gauge wire with a loop passed beneath the posterior

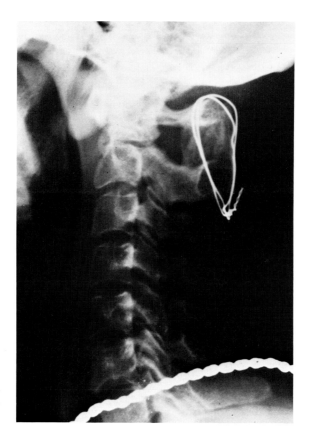

Figure 1–3E At 3 months there is solid fusion with complete recovery.

midline of C1; the loop is then brought over the spinous process of C2, with the two free ends of the wire then tightened beneath the spinous process of C2. An initial graft shaped like a pair of "hot pants" is combined with additional cancellous bone taken from the posterior iliac crest and placed beneath this wire (Figure 1–3E).

The type III fracture of the odontoid can be satisfactorily handled by the use of a halo vest, with an anticipated high rate of union (*1,7,22,24*).

The Hangman's fracture, whether it is associated with or without a fracture of the body of C2 and/or C3 (Figure 1–2C), can uniformly be treated closed (*21*) with a halo vest (*11*). We have seen no nonunions in 13 cases treated in this fashion (Table 1–1).

Any fracture at C4 or above, associated with a complete cord lesion, carries a poor prognosis; in such cases posterior stabilization for rapid mobilization of the patient to prevent the many complications seen with a prolonged recumbency may be indicated. We also do not quarrel with simple halo vest immobilization for this type of patient.

Mid and Lower Cervical Spine

We have defined specific fracture patterns that can be easily identified (Figures 1–1A, 1–2D–L, 1–3A). Here again, defining the neurologic deficit is paramount in the decision of whether to treat the patient with a closed or an open method and whether the anterior or posterior approach is utilized.

Cervical Spine Fractures

The commonly seen unilateral facet fracture and/or dislocation, if untreated, carries a high incidence of late cervical pain (35) and is frequently associated with significant nerve root impingement. In approximately 50% of our cases initially treated by closed methods, it was necessary later to carry out a posterior reduction, nerve root decompression, and posterior wire stabilization with cervical fusion. Because of this, if a patient presents with a significant nerve root involvement without cord involvement related to this injury, we prefer early posterior open reduction and stabilization (5) because the nerve can be easily decompressed via the posterior approach at the time of the operative procedure (Figures 1–2D–F). If the unilateral facet fracture and/or subluxation is without neurologic involvement, a halo vest is an alternative, nonsurgical modality of treatment.

A bilateral facet fracture dislocation is often associated with a complete or incomplete cord lesion (32). When there is an incomplete cord deficit, it seems necessary to obtain as rapid a reduction as possible. We have used the commonly accepted method of using closed skeletal traction with increasing weights (32). However, we much prefer an open reduction and posterior stabilization of this injury unless it reduces easily with minimal weight. In our opinion, regardless of the method of reduction, spinal fusion is usually indicated in this type of fracture (Figure 1–2G).

The flexion teardrop fracture dislocation/burst fracture with an incomplete cord syndrome presents a more difficult diagnostic and surgical problem. It may be associated with anterior and posterior column instability, and the anterior approach can compound this instability (3,34,36). Nevertheless, bony and/or disc fragments impinging on the anterior aspect of the spinal cord, with an anterior, central, or lateral cord syndrome, may demand an anterior approach for appropriate decompression (5). (We believe it is particularly unwise to treat an anterior cord compression syndrome with a posterior surgical approach.) For these problems, a fibular strut graft placed anteriorly after decompression has been strongly advocated by others (9). We prefer a tricortical graft taken from the anterior iliac crest at the time of anterior fusion. This graft is turned upside down, and sufficient bone is removed from each end that the graft resembles a rectangular hat. The graft is then inserted interlocking with the intact vertebra above and below the level of involvement (5). It is important to remove sufficient bone and disc fragments in order to totally decompress the anterior aspect of the cord to the posterior longitudinal ligament and/or dura prior to insertion of the graft. The use of the microscope has been a valuable adjunct. We rely on the neurosurgeon for this part of the procedure. (At times, an entire vertebral body must be removed for adequate decompression.)

We have not found it necessary to use additional internal fixation in the form of a plate (4,38) but believe that the immediate postoperative immobilization provided by the halo vest is mandatory. We have also not found it necessary to later combine a posterior approach with posterior stabilization to maintain stability (Figures 1–4A–D).

If there is a complete cord and an intact nerve root at the level of the injury, we prefer a simple posterior stabilization for rapid mobilization of the patient. If there are medical contraindications to surgery in the latter case, early application of a halo vest (5) is an alternative approach because healing usually occurs albeit with some residual deformity.

A degree of instability in a pure ligamentous injury frequently goes undetected. Therefore it is wise to obtain a supervised flexion and extension lateral view of the cervical spine if this is suspected (Figures 1–2I,J).

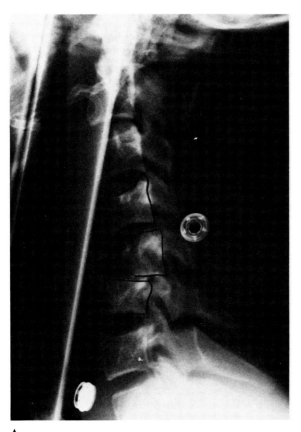 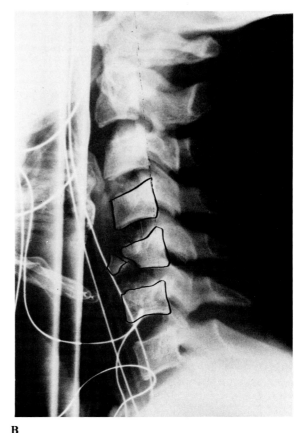

Figure 1–4 Flexion "teardrop" fracture dislocation/burst with a Brown-Sequard deficit in a 16-year-old male involved in an MVA. **A** Injury x-rays. **B** Gardner-Wells traction.

If there is pure posterior ligamentous disruption with a compression fracture, an inherently unstable injury (*34*), we prefer posterior fusion and wiring.

A lateral mass fracture is usually inherently stable and, for the most part, is treated by a closed method (Figures 1–2K,L).

Diagnostic Aids

There is no question that tomography of the cervical spine is a very useful tool for obtaining adequate detail of bony structural abnormalities. It is readily available in most institutions and is less complicated to carry out than CT scanning (Figures 1–2B,E–G,L). We also believe that myelography is extremely helpful in certain incomplete spinal cord syndromes and isolated nerve root impingements. A typical example is patient V.S., who presented with a classic Brown-Sequard syndrome secondary to a unilateral facet subluxation at C5–C6. It was decided to treat this injury in a closed fashion with preliminary skeletal traction; the result was an excellent reduction. A halo vest was then applied. The patient's neurologic condition plateaued, and at 3 weeks there was still a significant, persisting neurologic deficit. A myelogram done with the patient in the halo vest showed an obvious residual anterior compression defect. Anterior decompression and cervical fusion were done at this point with

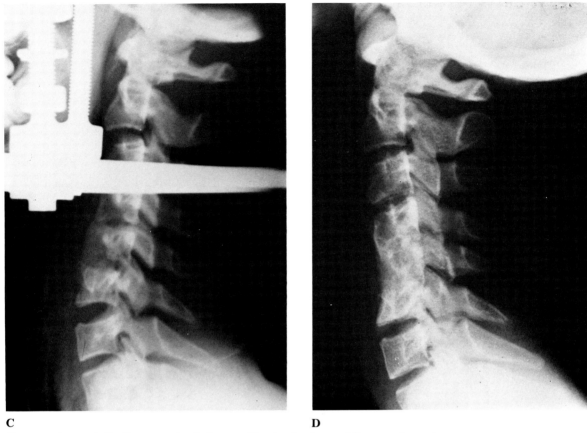

C D

Figure 1–4 (cont.) C Postoperative halo vest. D At the 8-year follow-up the patient is back to racing motorcycles without neurologic deficit.

almost immediate improvement in neurologic function (Figures 1–5A–D). At 6 months the patient was doing well (Figure 1–5E,5F).

We believe myelography is also mandatory in a patient who presents with a significant cord injury and/or a nerve root deficit, and whose plain x-rays and tomograms show no bony abnormality (Figures 1–6A–C). The CT scan may well eliminate some of our previous indications for Pantopaque myelography, but a CT scan without additional metrizamide has not been satisfactory for demonstrating significant compression defects resulting from soft tissue (intervertebral disc) impingement (37). Ideally, if myelography is done in unstable fracture dislocations of the cervical spine, it should be preceded by appropriate halo vest immobilization to prevent significant displacement of the fracture or dislocation at the time of this specialized procedure (Figures 1–7A,B).

Technical Considerations

Gardner-Wells Tongs

The use of Gardner-Wells tongs is a simple technique that provides initial stabilization and reduction of the injury and has, in our clinic, completely replaced the old Crutchfield and/or Vinkie tongs. We prefer this to the immediate application of a halo, which is more time-consuming in the emergency room.

14   Teipner et al

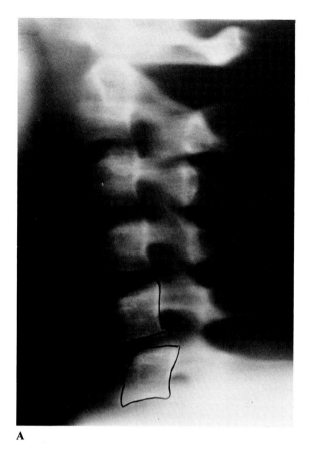

A

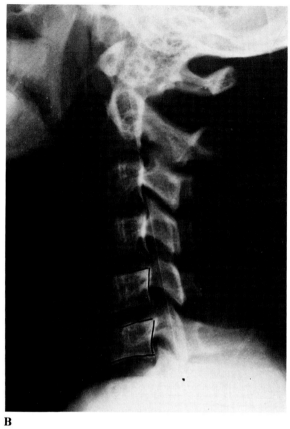

B

C

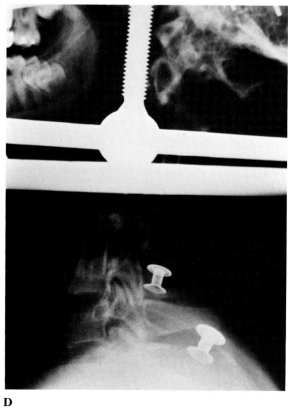

D

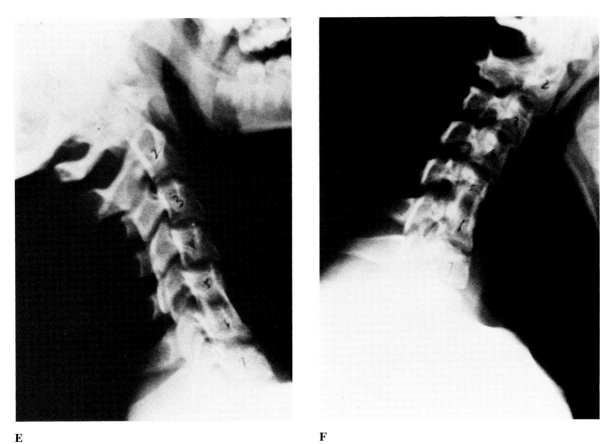

E   F

Figure 1–5 Unilateral facet dislocation with a Brown-Sequard deficit in a 13-year-old female involved in an MVA. **A** Tomogram of the unilateral facet dislocation. **B** Reduction in traction. **C** Myelogram 3 weeks after injury shows the reason for persistent neurologic deficit (*arrow*). **D** Decompression after an anterior strut graft with the patient in a halo vest. **E** At 6 months, extension and **F** at 6 months, flexion. The patient is ambulatory without external aids.

Halo and Halo Vest

A special head-holding device is useful to allow the application of a halo and halo vest with minimal assistance and minimal manipulation of the neck. Our own device was designed by our prosthetist Walter Benecke; it fits on the operating table, is easily adjustable, and does not have to be sterilized. Insertion of the posterior pins anywhere behind the ear presents no problem. Ideally, the anterior pins are placed above the outer canthus of the eye, but the alternative of placing them in the hairline, somewhat more posteriorly, is cosmetically more acceptable, particularly in a female patient.

The halo itself is placed 0.25 inch above the eyebrow and above the external ear. The immediate application of the vest at the time of halo application has allowed rapid mobilization of the patient regardless of the neurologic status and of whether a closed or open method of treatment has been selected.

Somi Brace and Philadelphia Collar

Other forms of postoperative immobilization are selected when indicated; for a stable posterior fusion we recommend a Somi brace during the day and a Philadelphia collar at night. The degree of patient compliance is often impor-

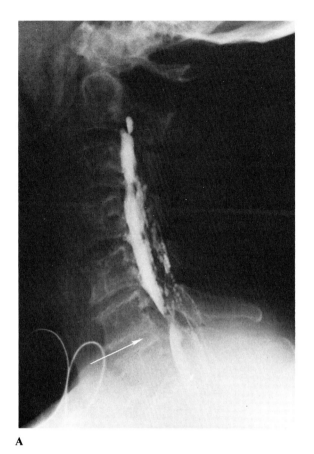

A

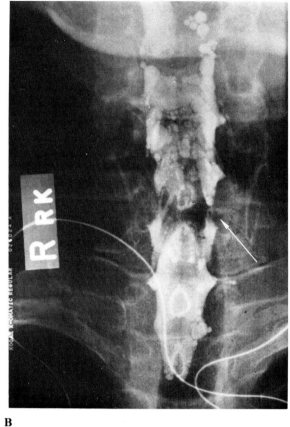

B

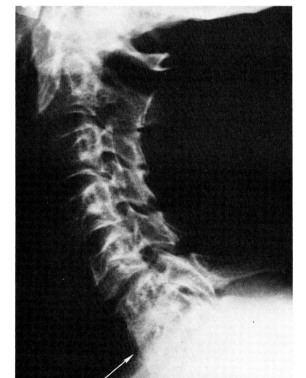

C

Figure 1–6 Disc protrusion with a Brown-Sequard deficit in a 43-year-old male involved in an MVA. **A** Lateral myelogram showing a C6–C7 disc protrusion (*arrow*). **B** Anteroposterior myelogram view of the disc protrusion (*arrow*). **C** At 3 months there is complete recovery after anterior decompression and fusion (*arrow*).

Cervical Spine Fractures

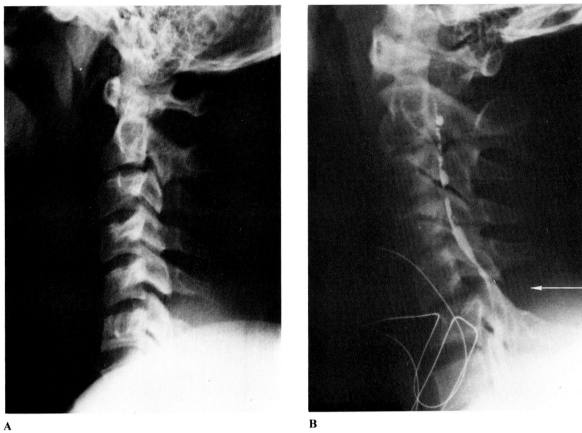

Figure 1-7 Posterior ligamentous disruption with an anterior cord syndrome in an 18-year-old male involved in an MVA. **A** Gardner-Wells traction. **B** Myelogram of the patient without halo vest immobilization. Note the redisplacement of the injury (*arrow*).

tant; and if we are concerned about this, particularly in patients among the younger age groups, we prefer the halo vest.

Urgency of Decompression

It is difficult to make a concrete statement regarding the urgency of decompression. The risk of early surgery must be weighed against the possible benefits, particularly in a freshly injured patient who frequently has other pressing injuries. There have been reports of a high morbidity and mortality rate among patients with complete cervical cord injuries treated by an early anterior approach (*18*). The anterior approach for this condition is used, presumably, for better nerve root decompression and better nerve root sparing.

Summary

Although the mechanism of injury is important, and granted that certain fracture types call for either closed or surgical treatment, the neurologic deficit is the deciding factor when selecting the appropriate treatment modality. The prime advantage of surgical treatment is prompt and thorough decompression of the cord or compromised nerve roots. Surgical decompression affords the significant added benefit of earlier mobilization of the patient toward a more meaningful existence. The use of prolonged recumbency with skeletal traction is not an attractive alternative in this era.

Acknowledgments

We wish to acknowledge the help and expertise of the following neurosurgeons: Charles E. Fleming, William N. Dawson Jr., Joseph R. Walker, John S. Davis, Ernest W. Mack, and Louis A. Levy; as well as physiatrists Walter J. Treanor and H. Haydon Hill.

REFERENCES

1. Anderson LD, D'Alonzo RT (1974). Fractures of the odontoid process of the axis. J Bone Joint Surg 56-A:1663–1674.
2. Bailey RW (1974). The Cervical Spine. Lea & Febiger, Philadelphia.
3. Bell GD, Bailey SI (1977). Section II. General orthopaedics: anterior cervical fusion for trauma. Clin Orthop 128:155–158.
4. Bohler J, Gaudenak T (1980). Anterior plate stabilization for fracture dislocations of the lower cervical spine. J Trauma 20:203–205.
5. Bohlman HH (1979). Acute fractures and dislocations of the cervical spine: an analysis of 300 hospitalized patients and review of the literature. J Bone Joint Surg 61A:1119–1124.
6. Cooper PR, Maravilla KR, Sklar FH, et al. (1979). Halo immobilization of cervical spine fractures: indications and results. J Neurosurg 50:603–610.
7. Ekong CE, Schwartz ML, Tator CH, et al. (1981). Odontoid fracture: management with early mobilization using the halo device. Neurosurgery 9:631–637.
8. Fielding JW (1973). The cervical spine in the child. In: Current Practice in Orthopaedic Surgery, Vol. 5, edited by Ahstrom JP Jr. Mosby, St. Louis.
9. Fielding JW, Rubin BD, Stillwell WT (1978). Cervical spine trauma. J Cont Educ Orthop July:19–31.
10. Fielding JW, Hensinger RN, Hawkins RJ (1980). Os odontoidium. J Bone Joint Surg 62A:376–383.
11. Francis WR, Fielding JW, Hawkins JR, et al. (1981). Traumatic spondylolisthesis of the axis. J Bone Joint Surg 63B:313–318.
12. Galli WE (1939). Fractures and dislocations of the cervical spine. Am J Surg 46:495.
13. Garber JN (1964). Abnormalities of the atlas and axis vertebrae—congenital and traumatic. J Bone Joint Surg 46A:1792.
14. Garber JN (1969). Fracture and fracture dislocation of the cervical spine. In: American Academy of Orthopaedic Surgeons: Symposium on the Spine. Mosby, St. Louis.
15. Han SY, Witten DM, Musselman JP (1976). Jefferson fracture of the atlas: report of six cases. J Neurosurg 44:368–371.
16. Hardy AG, Rossier AB (1975). Spinal Cord Injuries, edited by Thieme. Publishing Sciences Group, Acton, Mass.
17. Harris JH Jr (1978). The Radiology of Acute Cervical Spine Trauma. Williams & Wilkins, Baltimore.
18. Heiden JS, Weiss MH, Rosenberg AW, et al. (1975). Management of cervical spinal cord trauma in southern California. J Neurosurg 43:732–736.
19. Hoppenfeld S (1977). Orthopaedic Neurology. Lippincott, Philadelphia.
20. Jefferson G (1920). Fractures of the atlas vertebrae: report of four cases and review of those previously recorded. Br J Surg 7:407.
21. Pepin JW, Hawkins RJ (1981). Traumatic spondylolisthesis of the axis: hangman's fracture. Clin Orthop 157:133–138.

Cervical Spine Fractures

22. Ryan MD, Taylor TK (1982). Odontoid fractures: a rational approach to treatment. J Bone Joint Surg 64B:416–421.
23. Scher AT (1982). "Tear-drop" fractures of the cervical spine—radiological fractures. S Afr Med J 61:355–356.
24. Schiess RJ, DeSaussure RL, Robertson JT (1982). Choice of treatment of odontoid fractures. J Neurosurg 57:496–499.
25. Schneider RC (1951). A syndrome in acute cervical spine injuries for which early operation is indicated. J Neurosurg 8:360.
26. Schneider RC (1955). The syndrome of acute anterior cervical spinal cord injury. J Neurosurg 12:95–122.
27. Schneider RC, Cherry GL, Pantek HE (1954). The syndrome of acute central cervical spinal cord injury. J Neurosurg 11:546–577.
28. Schneider RC, Crosby EC, Russo RH, Gosch HH (1973). Traumatic spinal cord syndromes and their management. In: Clinical Neurosurgery, edited by Wilkins RH. Williams & Wilkins, Baltimore.
29. Schneider RC, Kahn EA (1956). Chronic neurologic sequelae of acute trauma to the spine and spinal cord. 1. The significance of the acute flexion or "tear-drop" fracture dislocation of the cervical spine. J Bone Joint Surg 38A:985–997.
30. Schneider RC, Livingston KE, Cave AJE, Hamilton G (1965). "Hangman's fracture" of the cervical spine. J Neurosurg 22:1412.
31. Shields CL Jr, Stauffer ES (1976). Late instability in cervical spine fractures secondary to laminectomy. Clin Orthop 76:144–147.
32. Sonntag VK (1981). Management of bilateral locked facets of the cervical spine. Neurosurgery 8:150–152.
33. Stauffer ES (1983). Personal communication.
34. Stauffer ES, Kelly EG (1977). Fracture dislocations of the cervical spine: instability and recurrent deformity following treatment by anterior interbody fusion. J Bone Joint Surg 59A:45–48.
35. Stauffer ES, Rhoades ME (1976). Surgical stabilization of the cervical spine after trauma. Arch Surg 111:652–657.
36. Van Peteghem PK, Schweigel JF (1979). The fractured cervical spine rendered unstable by anterocervical fusion. J Trauma 19:110–114.
37. Virapongse C, Wagner F Jr, Sarwar M, Kier EL (1983). The choice of contrast agent for myelography in patients with nonpenetrating cervical spine trauma. Radiology 147:465–471.
38. Waisbrod H (1981). Anterior cervical spine fusion for unstable fractures. Injury 12:389–392.
39. Zimmerman E, Grant J, Vise WM, et al. (1976). Treatment of Jefferson fractures with a halo apparatus: report of two cases. J Neurosurg 44:372–375.

Supracondylar and Intercondylar Fractures of the Adult Humerus

2

Marshall Horowitz

Fractures of the distal end of the humerus are not common; hence no one method of treatment has evolved which is superior to others and acceptable to all who treat these difficult fractures. Riseborough and Radin (*10*) and the Swiss Association for the Study of Internal Fixation (*8,9*) have identified several recurring fracture patterns. The supracondylar fracture occurs within an area of approximately 4–5 cm proximal to the upper border of the olecranon. The fracture is either transverse or short oblique and may be slightly comminuted (Figure 2–1). There is, however, no intraarticular involvement. Intercondylar fractures are most often referred to as T-type or Y-type fractures. The capitellum and trochlea are displaced and/or rotated (Figure 2–2). In the most severe type, there is considerable comminution of the articular surfaces of the capitellum and trochlea, the olecranon fossa, and the adjacent metaphyseal-diaphyseal region otherwise identified as the medial and lateral epicondylar ridges. Depending on the degree of violence, some of these fractures may be open (Figure 2–3). Vehicular accidents and falls from heights on the flexed elbow account for most of these injuries. The fractures may be isolated or associated with other orthopaedic injuries in the polytraumatized patient.

A retrospective review of surgically treated fractures of the distal end of the humerus was performed between 1973 and 1983. Experience in the application of improved surgical implants and techniques enhanced our ability to treat these fractures more adequately than in prior years. The evolution of treatment was no different in our patient population than is reported in the literature (*7*). Manipulations and long arm casts yielded to olecranon pin traction, early motion, and long arm casts. Motion within a serviceable range was the exception rather than the rule. Operative treatment with less than optimal fixation was at times worse than nonoperative treatment. Operative success was not guaranteed if even the most sophisticated surgical implants were applied inappropriately (Figure 2–4).

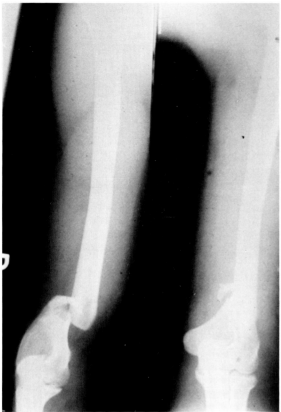 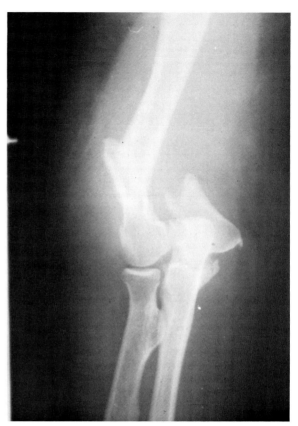

Figure 2–1 Short-oblique, comminuted supracondylar fracture of the humerus.

Figure 2–2 Displaced, rotated T-condylar fracture of the humerus.

The department of orthopaedic surgery at our institution reviewed 25 supracondylar and intercondylar fractures of the humerus in 24 patients treated by open reduction and internal fixation. Eighteen fractures were closed injuries, and seven were open; of the seven open fractures, three were the result of gunshot wounds. One patient had bilateral fractures, a supracondylar fracture of one extremity, and a comminuted T-condylar fracture of the other. There were 12 males and 12 females ranging in age from 14 to 55 years. Extremity function was evaluated with regard to elbow flexion and extension, forearm supination and pronation, and the patient's subjective symptoms. The result was rated excellent, good, fair, or poor according to a slight modification of the criteria set forth by Riseborough and Radin (*10*).

Operative Technique

Preoperative evaluation of the patient and planning of the operative procedure are essential. In order to adequately visualize the distal end of the humerus, the position of the patient must allow 120° of elbow flexion during the operative procedure. The patient may be placed in either the prone or the lateral position. A pneumatic tourniquet is placed around the upper arm and inflated after prepping and draping the extremity. The incision begins in the midline of the arm approximately 12–15 cm proximal to the tip of the olecranon; it is carried distally and slightly lateral to the olecranon, and then distally along the subcuta-

Humeral Fractures

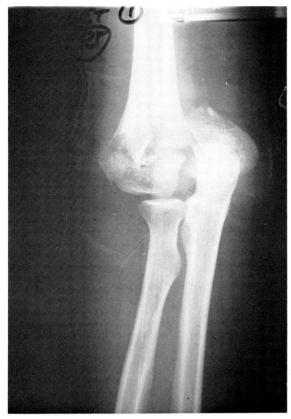

Figure 2–3 Open, comminuted T-condylar fracture of the humerus.

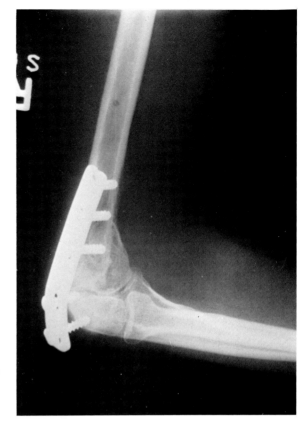

Figure 2–4 Inappropriate application of a broad DC plate.

neous border of the ulna for another 5–7 cm. Medial and lateral skin flaps are elevated exposing the triceps aponeurosis proximally (Figure 2–5) and the olecranon and proximal antebrachial fascia distally. The ulnar nerve *must* be identified before proceeding any further. A Penrose drain about the nerve aids in identifying the nerve throughout the operative procedure.

Supracondylar and T- and Y-condylar fractures of the humerus are most frequently and adequately exposed by utilizing the Campbell approach (*13*). Fractures with considerable comminution of the capitellum and trochlea are exposed by osteotomy of the olecranon, as described by Cassebaum (*4,5*).

Campbell Exposure of the Humerus

A tongue of triceps aponeurosis is sharply developed beginning at the level of the proximal extent of the skin incision and is extended distally and based on the medial and lateral borders of the olecranon. Hematoma within the triceps musculature and/or laceration of the muscle leads the way through the triceps in the midline to the humerus. Hematoma is removed as encountered, and with a periosteal elevator the musculature is elevated from the posteromedial and posterolateral aspects of the proximal humerus fragment. Medial and lateral retractors are inserted with care, and undue force is avoided during exposure because intraoperative traction injuries to the radial nerve do occur occasionally (Figure 2–6).

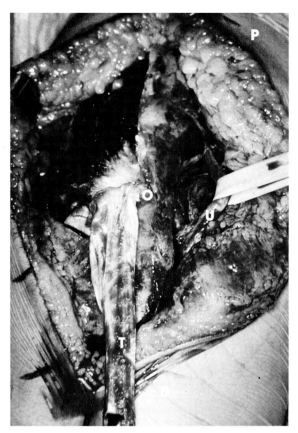 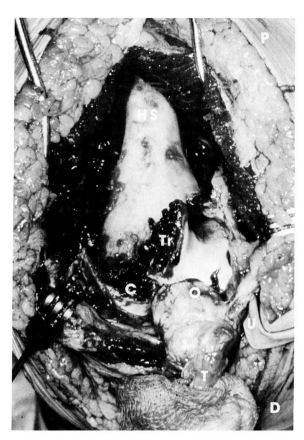

Figure 2–5 Exposure of the ulnar nerve and distal reflection of the triceps aponeurosis. (*P*) proximal. (*D*) distal. (*U*) ulnar nerve. (*T*) triceps aponeurosis. (*O*) olecranon.

Figure 2–6 Campbell exposure of a T-condylar fracture of the humerus. (*P*) proximal. (*D*) distal. (*U*) ulnar nerve. (*T*) triceps aponeurosis. (*O*) olecranon. (*HS*) humeral shaft. (*C*) capitellum. (*Tr*) trochlea.

Cassebaum Exposure of the Humerus

The soft tissues medial and lateral to the olecranon are sharply elevated, and a thin osteotome is utilized to divide the olecranon 0.5–1.0 cm proximal to the coronoid process. Care must be taken to avoid injury to the ulnar nerve. Prior to performing the osteotomy, a 3.2-mm hole is drilled through the tip of the olecranon and into the proximal ulna to facilitate its repair after fixation of the humerus is completed. The osteotome should be driven just below the level of the articular surface. The latter is cracked by using the osteotome as a lever. This precludes inadvertent penetration of the osteotome into the already damaged humeral condyles. Once the olecranon has been osteotomized, it is reflected proximally while the triceps musculature is incised medially and laterally in a cephalad direction. The disrupted humeral condyles and the shaft of the humerus are readily visualized (Figure 2–7). Having divided the olecranon, it no longer serves as a template against which the comminuted articular surface can be molded.

Internal Fixation of Supracondylar Fractures

Supracondylar fractures are most easily exposed by the posterior Campbell approach. Most are transverse or short oblique fractures with minimal or no commi-

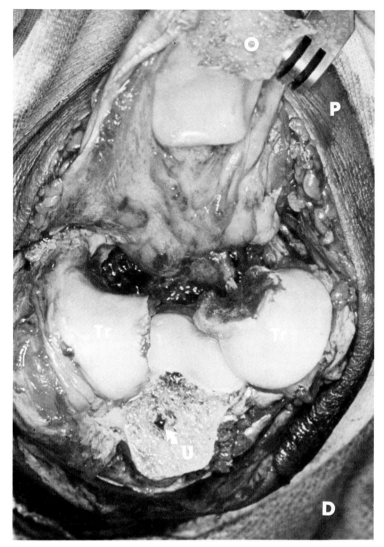
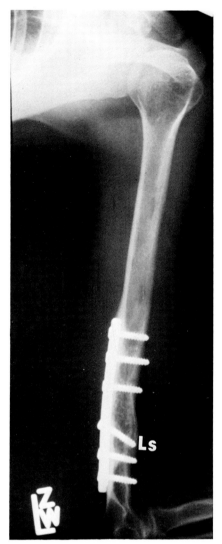

Figure 2–7 Cassebaum olecranon osteotomy. (*P*) proximal. (*D*) distal. (*U, arrow*) proximal ulna with drill hole. (*O*) osteotomized olecranon. (*Tr*) fractured trochlea.

Figure 2–8 Contoured broad DC plate with a lag screw (*Ls*).

nution; they may extend 4–5 cm proximal to the upper border of the olecranon fossa. The fragments are manipulated and the reduction temporarily maintained with reduction forceps and K-wires. A broad dynamic compression plate may be applied to the posterior surface of the humerus only if six distal cortices secure the plate to bone and the plate's distal extent does not project into the olecranon fossa, interfering with the excursion of the olecranon. Before its application, the plate must be contoured to the slightly convex posterior surface of the humerus. Proximally, six cortices suffice to secure the plate to the humerus (Figure 2–8). Tension can be applied across transverse or short oblique fracture fragments by employing the DC mechanism inherent in the plate. A screw inserted through a hole made with the "neutral drill guide" fixes the plate to bone; a second screw on the opposite side of the fracture is inserted into a hole made with the "load guide." As the screw is tightened, compression is produced between the fracture fragments, and any remaining fracture gap is obliterated. The remaining screws are inserted in the neutral position. Utilizing

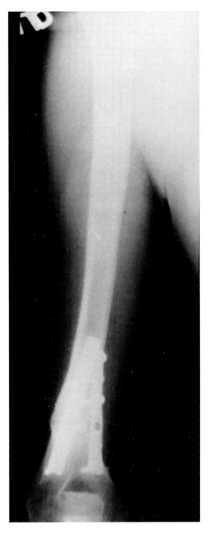

Figure 2–9 Dual posterior medial and lateral one-third tubular plates.

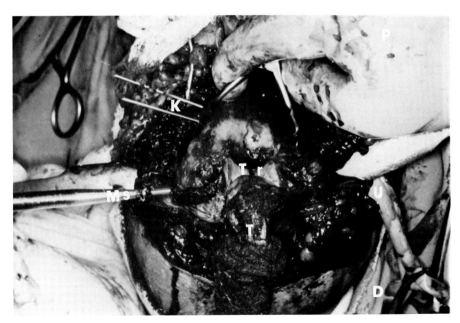

Figure 2–10 Reduction and fixation of condyles. (*P*) proximal. (*D*) distal. (*U*) ulnar nerve. (*T*) triceps aponeurosis. (*Tr*) reduced trochlea. (*K*) K-wires. (*Ms*) malleolar screw.

the lag screw technique for cortical screws, interfragmentary compression can be accomplished, if possible. A broad DC plate is selected because the screw holes are alternately offset from center, precluding propagation of linear fracture lines as might occur with a narrow DC plate.

An alternative method of fixation may be employed when the distal segment is short and will not accept a posteriorly placed broad DC plate. Posterolateral and posteromedial one-third tubular or 3.5-mm DC plates offer an excellent means of internal fixation in this instance. Each plate is secured to the distal fragment with a minimum of two to three 3.5-mm cortical screws. Proximally, at least three bicortical screws must secure each plate to bone (Figure 2–9).

Internal Fixation of Intercondylar Fractures

T- and Y-intercondylar fractures without comminution are accessible by the Campbell posterior approach. Severely comminuted fractures should be exposed by olecranon osteotomy as described previously. Regardless of the fracture type, the congruity of the articular surface must be reestablished. The capitellum and trochlea in T- and Y-fractures are reduced and temporarily stabilized with a Kirschner wire(s). Definitive fixation is obtained with a cancellous-type screw usually inserted from the lateral side (Figure 2–10). Comminuted fractures may require Kirschner wires in addition to a cancellous screw in order to restore the articular surface and block rotation of the fragments. Butterfly fragments along the epicondylar ridges are reattached to the shaft with lag screws. The reassembled humeral condyles are now reduced to the shaft, and continuity between the two is reestablished with posteromedial and posterolateral plates (Figure 2–11). Contoured one-third tubular or 3.5-mm DC plates are most

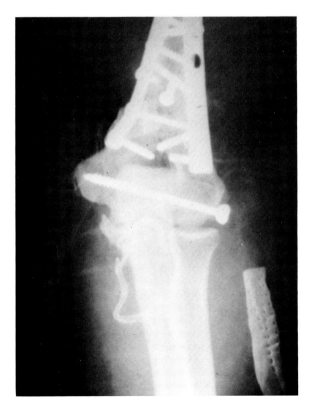

Figure 2–11 Repaired T-condylar fracture (see text).

commonly utilized. Care must be taken to avoid encroachment of the olecranon fossa by implants and bone debris. Visual inspection and intraoperative radiographs determine the alignment, and motion of the elbow indicates ease of movement and stability of fixation. Defects or comminution may require an autogenous cancellous iliac bone graft.

Repair of an Olecranon Osteotomy

To repair an olecranon osteotomy a 2.0-mm drill hole is made transversely through the ulna distal to the osteotomy site. The distance should be equal to the length of the previously osteotomized olecranon. The olecranon is reduced to the shaft and stabilized with a 6.5-mm cancellous screw and washer inserted through the 3.2-mm hole drilled prior to osteotomy. A length of 18-gauge wire is placed through the transverse drill hole, looped around the screw head and washer in a figure-of-eight fashion, and tightened (Figure 2–12). The ulnar nerve may be transferred anteriorly if the surgical implants encroach on its bed.

Soft tissues are drained, and the incision is closed in layers. A Robert-Jones bandage is applied with the elbow at 90° of flexion. The incisions are inspected at 3–5 days postoperatively, and gentle active motion may be initiated at this time. During periods of inactivity, the extremity is splinted and elevated. In instances where rigid stabilization has been compromised by comminution or osseous defects, an orthosis may be fabricated to support the extremity, or the extremity may be immobilized in a long arm cast for approximately 3 weeks.

Results

Two of seven patients with supracondylar fractures of the humerus had associated ipsilateral forearm fractures. One patient had segmental fractures of the radius and ulna. A second patient had a fracture of the olecranon and proximal radius.

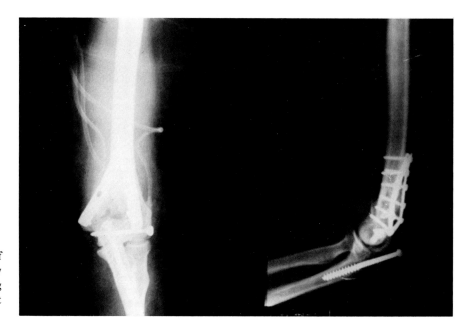

Figure 2–12 Repair of an olecranon osteotomy with a cancellous lag screw and figure-of-eight wire.

Humeral Fractures

Four patients had isolated supracondylar humerus fractures, and one patient had fractures of all four extremities, including a contralateral comminuted, T-condylar fracture. Of the seven supracondylar fractures, two were open and isolated injuries. In five instances a single broad DC plate was used, and in two medial and lateral one-third tubular plates were used. Both ipsilateral forearm fractures were treated with internal fixation at the time the humerus was repaired. The results were excellent in all seven supracondylar humerus fractures. The four patients with isolated fractures had normal elbow extension and flexion. Forearm supination-pronation was unimpaired, and the patients were functionally no different from their preinjury status. A similar result was obtained with the extremity of the patient who had fractured all four extremities. One of the patients with an associated ipsilateral forearm fracture had unrestricted elbow and forearm function, but the patient with the associated olecranon and radius fracture lacked 20° of extension and 20° of pronation (Figure 2–13). Two radial nerve palsies occurred among this group of fractures. One was undetected preoperatively, and subsequent clinical and electrodiagnostic studies revealed no evidence of functional return of radial nerve activity. Appropriate tendon transfers were performed at 5 months after injury. One intraoperatively occurring radial nerve palsy fully recovered after 16 weeks.

A 14-year-old male had a displaced, nonrotated T-condylar fracture of the humerus. Intraarticular congruency was reestablished with a cancellous lag screw, and the reassembled condyles were secured to the shaft with contoured medial and lateral one-third tubular plates. Normal function was achieved.

Eight T- and Y-condylar fractures were both displaced and rotated. All had three major fragments—the shaft, trochlea, and capitellum—and were without significant comminution. Treatment was similar in all cases: After restoring the articular surface with a 4.0-mm cancellous lag screw or a 4.5-mm malleolar screw, the reassembled trochlea and capitellum were secured to the shaft with either two contoured one-third tubular plates or a one-third tubular and 3.5-mm DC plate.

Results were excellent in five fractures with normal elbow flexion-extension and forearm supination-pronation. There were no subjective complaints of pain or weakness. The patient whose injury resulted from a gunshot wound lost 15° of forearm pronation and 30° of supination. He lacked the last 30° of elbow extension and could flex to 120°. He complained of mild pain and some weakness, but his result was considered good. One extremity was considered fair because elbow flexion-extension, although within a serviceable range, was less than 90°. Supination-pronation were restricted by 20° in each plane. The elbow lacked the last 40° of full extension but would flex to 120°. Pain and weakness accompanied the lost motion. Fixation failed in one patient, although the fracture united after immobilization in an orthosis. Although the elbow lacked 30° of extension, 90° of flexion was achieved. Supination and pronation were limited by 30° in each direction. The patient complained of pain and weakness as well and was considered to have a poor result.

There were nine comminuted fractures of the distal end of the humerus. Of four open fractures, two were the result of gunshot wounds. Treatment of these fractures differed only in that articular restoration was more difficult, necessitating the use of screws and K-wires. Bone defects were grafted and bridged with medial and lateral contoured plates. There were no excellent results in this group of patients. Four elbows were considered "good" in that elbow flexion-extension averaged slightly better than 90° and forearm pronation-supination was not restricted more than 20° in either plane, except in one patient whose fracture was the result of a gunshot wound. Complaints of pain and

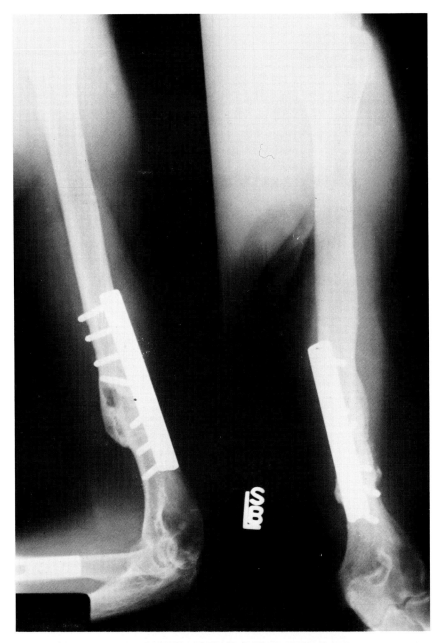

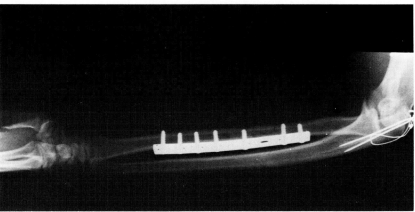

Figure 2–13 Internal fixation of the ipsilateral humerus, olecranon, and radius fracture.

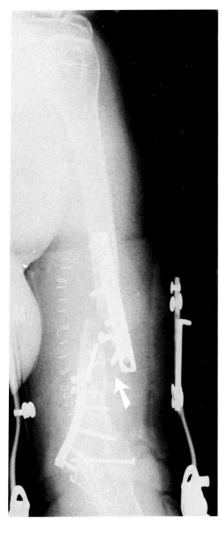

Figure 2–14 Failure of fixation and refracture of the shaft (*arrow*).

weakness were minimal. There were two fair results. One patient lacked 50° of elbow extension and could flex an additional 70°. Pain and weakness were constant complaints. A severely comminuted open fracture with an associated preoperative radial nerve palsy in a 55-year-old female was immobilized in an orthosis after the shaft refractured between a distal medial and proximal lateral plate (Figure 2–14). Complete radial nerve function returned after 8 weeks, and subsequently the fracture united at 16 weeks after injury. The elbow lacked 15° of extension and would flex to 110°. Forearm supination and pronation were limited by 15° in each plane. Although pain was not a symptom, the patient complained of slight weakness. Overall, the result was considered fair because the goals of internal fixation were not achieved. Of the three poor results, one was from a gunshot wound; a second occurred after a one-third tubular plate failed; and the third occurred after inadequate internal fixation. In the latter fracture, minimal and inadequate internal fixation necessitated external immobilization in a long arm cast. The elbow became ankylosed at 90° and in neutral forearm rotation. The patient whose plate failed is still being treated for the resultant nonunion. The gunshot injury caused significant loss of elbow function. Elbow extension and flexion were limited to an arc of 60°, between 50° and 110° of flexion. Forearm rotation was no greater than 10° in either direction.

Briefly, seven supracondylar fractures of the humerus alone or with associated ipsilateral forearm fractures had excellent functional results after internal fixation. Of nine T- and Y-intercondylar fractures, six were considered excellent, one good, one fair, and one poor. There were no excellent results in the nine comminuted fractures. There were four good, two fair, and three poor extremities.

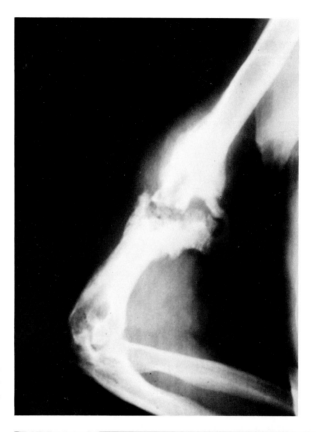

Figure 2–15A Infected nonunion. Failure of fixation, infection, and nonunion.

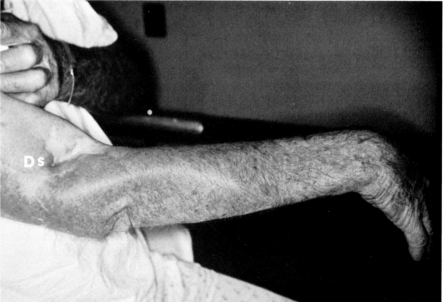

Figure 2–15B Infected non-union. Radial nerve palsy and a lacerated brachial artery. (*D*s) draining sinus.

Humeral Fractures
33

Complications

When considering operative treatment for fractures of the distal end of the humerus, the complications of such treatment, which are significant and serious, must be borne in mind. They are best illustrated in a patient seen in consultation. In an effort to salvage an infected nonunion after internal fixation, the radial nerve and brachial artery were transected (Figures 2–15A,B).

There were no infections in our series. Failure of fixation, which occurred in three instances, was thought to have resulted from overbending a plate through a screw hole on two occasions and through an area of increased stress between a medially and laterally positioned plate in another. Of these failures of fixation, one required reoperation for nonunion, whereas two eventually healed after immobilization in an orthosis. Failure of fixation in these three patients compromised the final functional result, with one fair and two poor results.

There were three radial nerve palsies. Two were present preoperatively. One occurred during the operative procedure, no doubt caused by overzealous retraction during exposure and/or plate application. In the latter case, radial nerve function returned after 16 weeks. One preoperative palsy patient recovered after 8 weeks, whereas the second required appropriate tendon transfers to restore function. Because the ulnar nerve was always identified prior to exposure of the fracture, in no case did it sustain any injury.

Discussion

Fractures of the distal end of the humerus have been classified by Riseborough and Radin (*10*) and Mueller et al. (*9*) into supracondylar and T- and Y-condylar fractures. Although the classification remains constant, methods of treatment vary considerably. Nonoperative treatment consisting of manipulation or skeletal traction with subsequent cast immobilization has been advocated by some (*7,10*). Still others recommend open reduction and internal fixation as the optimum method of treatment (*1–5,7–9,12*).

During the past 10 years, we have recognized an evolution in treatment. As noted above, closed reduction and cast immobilization preceded skeletal traction and "early motion," which in turn yielded to early internal fixation. Prolonged immobilization has a deleterious effect on normal articular surfaces (*6,11*), and Salter and Ogilvie-Harris (*11*) recently showed that injured articular cartilage recovers more rapidly and better when anatomically repaired, stabilized, and placed in motion. Hence it seems that open reduction and internal fixation, particularly in articular injuries, is a reasonable approach to these injuries.

Supracondylar fractures of the humerus require internal fixation when closed reduction can be neither achieved nor maintained. Similarly, to facilitate early extremity function, those humerus fractures which are associated with ipsilateral forearm fractures should be surgically stabilized. Operative treatment should also be considered in patients with bilateral humeral fractures and those persons sustaining multiple trauma. In the latter instances, the ease in nursing, patient comfort, and early extremity motion enhance the patient's overall rehabilitation. All seven patients whose supracondylar fractures and ipsilateral forearm fractures were treated with internal fixation had excellent functional results.

Among the group of nine patients with displaced and rotated intraarticular fractures of the distal end of the humerus, there were only two less than satisfactory results. Immobilization in an orthosis was required in one patient after one plate broke. Although a second patient's fracture healed without incident, total motion of the elbow was less than 90°.

There were five less than satisfactory results in the severely comminuted intraarticular fractures of the distal end of the humerus. A gunshot wound accounted for one poor result, and failures of internal fixation were responsible for one fair and one poor result. Although two fractures in this grouping united without incident, their ranges of motion were less than satisfactory, and the results were rated fair or poor.

Supracondylar and a majority of displaced and rotated intraarticular fractures of the humerus are amenable to internal fixation with anticipated good to excellent results. Those fractures of the distal end of the humerus with significant comminution can be surgically repaired with the expectation that good results can be obtained only if articular congruency can be restored, stable fixation is achieved, and a program of rehabilitation is followed.

REFERENCES

1. Bickel WE, Perry RE (1963). Comminuted fractures of the distal humerus. JAMA 184:553–557.
2. Bryan RS (1981). Fractures about the elbow in adults. In: Instructional Course Lectures, the American Academy of Orthopaedic Surgeons, Vol. 30. Mosby, St. Louis, pp. 200–223.
3. Bryan RS, Bickel MH (1971). "T" condylar fractures of the distal humerus. J Trauma 11:830–835.
4. Cassebaum WH (1952). Operative treatment of T and Y fractures of the lower end of the humerus. Am J Surg 83:265–270.
5. Cassebaum WH (1969). Open reduction of T and Y fractures of the lower end of the humerus. J Trauma 9:915–925.
6. Enneking WF, Horowitz M (1972). The intra-articular effects of immobilization on the human knee. J Bone Joint Surg 54A:973–985.
7. Eppright RH, Wilkens KE (1975). Fractures and dislocations of the elbow. In: Fractures, edited by Rockwood CA Jr, Green DP. Lippincott, Philadelphia, pp. 487–509.
8. Heim U, Pfeiffer KM (1974). The elbow. In: Small Fragment Set Manual. Springer-Verlag, New York, pp. 57–83.
9. Mueller ME, Allgoewer M, Schneider R, Willenegger H (1979). Fractures of the distal humerus. In: Manual of Internal Fixation, 2nd ed. Springer-Verlag, New York, pp. 176–181.
10. Riseborough EJ, Radin EL (1969). Intercondylar T-fractures of the humerus in the adult. J Bone Joint Surg 51A:130–141.
11. Salter RB, Ogilvie-Harris DJ (1979). Healing of intra-articular fractures with continuous passive motion. In: Instructional Course Lectures, the American Academy of Orthopaedic Surgeons, Vol. 28. Mosby, St. Louis, pp. 102–117.
12. Scharplatz D, Allgoewer M (1975). Fracture-dislocation of the elbow. Injury 7:143–159.
13. Sisk DS (1980). Fractures. In: Campbell's Operative Orthopaedics, Vol. 1, edited by Edmonson AS, Crenshaw AH. Mosby, St. Louis, pp. 674–679.

Small ASIF External Fixator for Fractures of the Wrist and Further Applications

3

Roland P. Jakob

The technical difficulties in the treatment of comminuted fractures of the distal radius by the usual techniques are obvious by the numerous unsatisfactory results. Closed reduction with plaster fixation is often complicated by a marked shortening even if accessory percutaneous Kirschner wire fixation is used. Surgical techniques of internal fixation are difficult. Open reduction of the impacted comminuted radial epiphysis and metaphysis demands an extensive soft tissue detachment. Because of the insufficient holding power of the screws, the risk of secondary displacement is marked. Application of a dorsal plate inhibits the free function of the extensor tendons.

Following Anderson and his methods of treatment of fractures of the distal radius (1), several authors recently have similarly recommended distraction of the wrist joint in an external fixator (1,2,4,5,9). The method is based on the observation that the length of the radius, restored by closed reduction, can be maintained by distraction because of the pull of the intact capsular ligamentous apparatus. This has been called "ligamentotaxis" by Vidal et al. (8).

For 5 years the small AO external fixator has produced good results and can be recommended in the treatment of the following fractures:

1. Unstable fractures of the distal radius
   Epiphyseal/metaphyseal comminution
   Metaphyseal comminution with loss of substance and massive dorsal tilt (Colles) or with marked radial shortening
   Fracture with volar tilt (Smith) or with volar intraarticular fragment (reversed Barton)
   Open fracture
   Comminuted fracture in combination with other fractures of the upper extremity or injuries of the hand

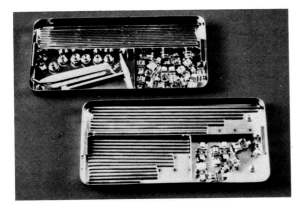
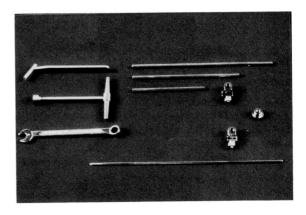

Figure 3–1 Instruments.

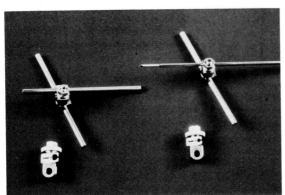

2. Fracture dislocations of the wrist joint
    Intraarticular comminuted fracture of the base of the first metacarpal
    Complex injuries of the hand where skeletal stabilization is not otherwise possible

Instruments

Instruments are kept in a small aluminium case, with two trays. The upper tray contains threaded K-wires 2.5/150 mm, clamps ϕ 4.0/2.5 mm, a combination wrench 7 mm, a socket wrench 7 mm, and a drill sleeve ϕ 2.5 mm. The lower tray contains clamps ϕ 4.0/4.0 mm, springloaded nuts (for quick temporary digital fixation), and connecting bars 60–200 mm (Figure 3–1). The contents can provide at least three or four different fixations. Additionally required are a small air drill with Jacob's chuck and key and a large wire cutter.

Surgical Technique

Standard Fixation With the Wrist Joint in a Neutral Position

Radius–Second Metacarpal Fixation in Unstable Fracture of the Distal Radius Using sterile conditions and the image intensifier, the fracture is manually reduced under an axillary block. Intraarticular fracture lines can be secured by percutaneous Kirschner wire fixation. If distraction alone does not result in a satisfactory position because articular fragments are too displaced or im-

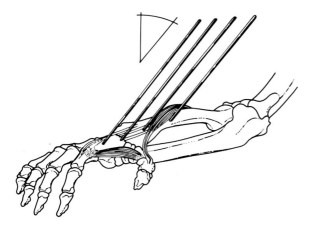

Figure 3–2 Insertion of wires.

pacted, reduction can be achieved by levering with percutaneous Kirschner wires or by open reduction. In young patients with a marked cancellous defect, an additional cancellous bone graft may be needed.

After making 5-mm incisions, the 2.5-mm threaded wires are inserted with the small air drill using a 2.5-mm tissue sleeve to protect the soft tissues. Two threaded K-wires are inserted proximal to the fracture in the radius, and two are inserted distally in the shaft of the second metacarpal. Sliding of the wires must be avoided. Maintaining the forearm and hand in pronation, the wires are inserted at an angle of 45° to both the horizontal and vertical planes, avoiding the extensor tendons. In the forearm the first wire is placed proximal to the palpable wad of the extensor pollicis brevis muscle and the abductor pollicis longus muscle. The distal wire is inserted between the tendons of the extensor carpi radialis brevis and longus muscles (Figure 3-2).

When inserting the wires in the metacarpal, the metacarpal-phalangeal joint is flexed to a right angle to avoid the extensor hood. The thumb is held in abduction to avoid the first web space (Figure 3-3).

Both proximally and distally, the two Kirschner wires must be inserted converging at an angle of 40°–60° in the bone, the points not touching each other. This allows a longer passage through the bone and thus more stable fixation, which is important in the second metacarpal. Each wire must obtain purchase in both cortices.

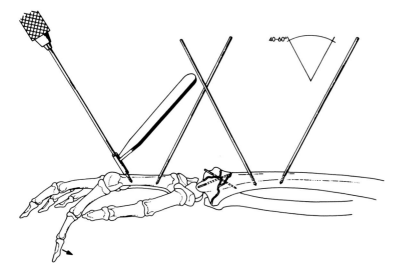

Figure 3–3 Insertion of wires prescribing an angle of 40°–60° within the same bow.

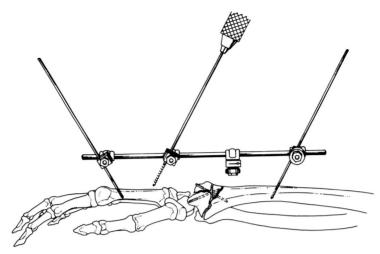

Figure 3–4 Application of manual clamps.

The two outer wires are drilled first, and the connecting rod is temporarily fixed. Placing the inner two wires is then facilitated by using the two inner loosely attached 4.0/2.5 mm clamps as aiming devices. The special manual clamps are applied to both threaded wires in the radius (Figure 3–4).

After application of the first rod adjacent to the bone, the two distal metacarpal clamps are fixed. Pulling on the fingers provides distraction. If the reduction under image intensifier is satisfactory, the proximal clamps with spring-loaded nuts are tightened manually. During this phase any change of position can be easily accomplished (Figure 3–5).

When adequate distraction and manipulation provide the desired reduction and maintenance of the fracture, a second rod is applied 2–3 cm further along the threaded wires. It serves mainly to neutralize the rotational forces. Finally, the special proximal manual clamps can be replaced by the definitive clamps (Figure 3–6). The advantages of this method are: a simple frame, ease of application, economical use of material, and stable fixation. A clinical example can be seen in Figure 3–7.

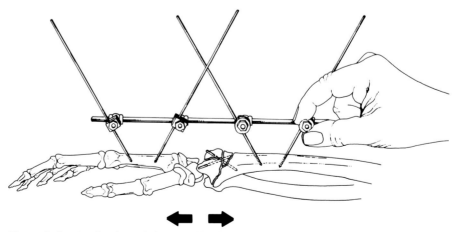

Figure 3–5 Application of the two distal metacarpal clamps.

Wrist Fractures

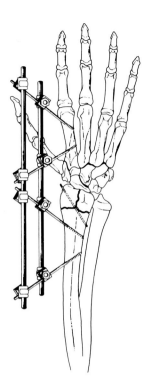

Figure 3–6 Application of a second rod.

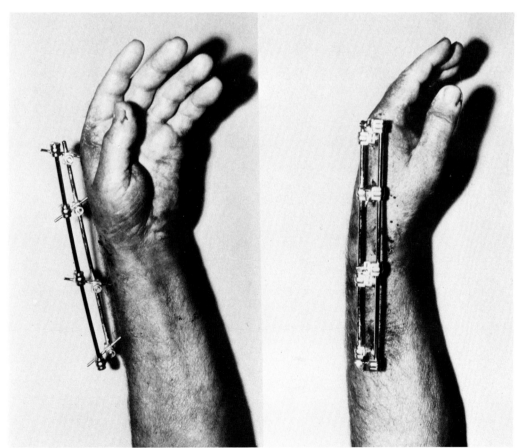

A

Figure 3–7 Clinical example of the standard radius–second metacarpal fixation for a distal fracture of the radius with a volar tilt (reversed Barton). An external fixator was applied for 7 weeks. There was a good result after 1 year.

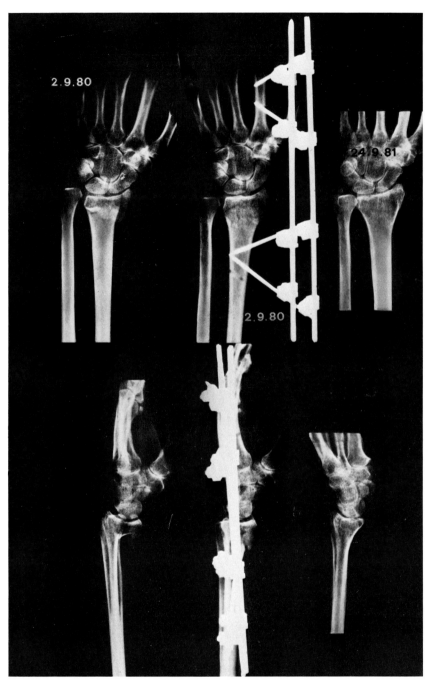

Figure 3–7 (cont.) B

Wrist Fractures

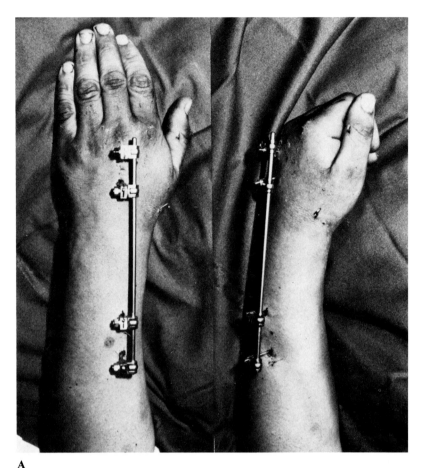

A

Figure 3–8 Complex perilunar fracture dislocation. Note the open reduction and Kirschner wire fixation from the volar side. Reduction is facilitated, after distraction, with the external fixator.

Fixation of the Radius to the Third Metacarpal in Fracture Dislocations of the Wrist Joint The advantage of using this method (Figure 3–8) is that there is a strictly neutral distraction without radial or ulnar deviation. The disadvantage is that there is impairment of the function of the extensor mechanism.

Distraction in Any Desired Position of the Wrist Joint

In Figure 3–9 it can be seen that each K-wire couple is fixed by two short rods. The desired position is then maintained by joining the proximal and distal short rods, under distraction, with 4.0/4.0 clamps. The advantages to this procedure are that fixation can be accomplished in any desired position of the wrist joint, and it can be used when only short rods are available. A clinical example may be seen in Figure 3–10.

Frame Fixation Without Crossing the Wrist Joint

Frame fixation without crossing the wrist joint is possible only when the distal articular fragment is not fractured and the osseous quality is good. Two

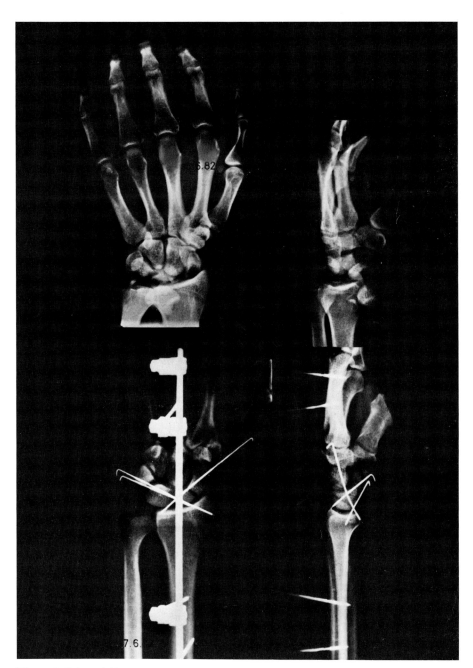

Figure 3–8 (cont.) B

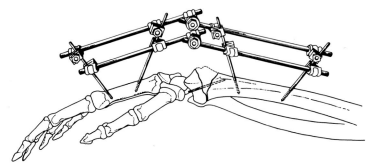

Figure 3–9 Distraction in any desired position.

Wrist Fractures

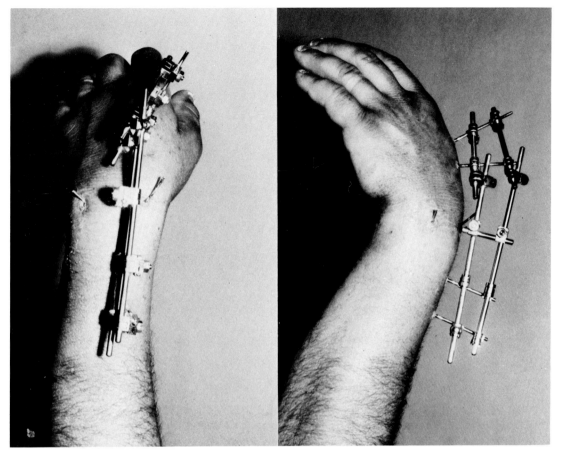

Figure 3–10 Distal fracture of the radius with dorsal comminution (Colles). Kirschner wire fixation alone did not suffice to stabilize the fracture. Almost anatomic reduction of the fracture was obtained with distraction and marked flexion of the wrist joint. After 3 weeks realignment of the wrist joint from flexion to a neutral position was performed. At 1 year after operation there was a good result.

wires are inserted parallel to the articular surface, one from the radial direction and the other from the dorsal direction into the distal fragment. They are then connected to a rectangular frame, under slight compression, to the proximal wires (Figure 3–11). The advantages of the method are that it provides a direct hold on the distal fragment and allows free mobility of the wrist joint. Its disadvantage is that there is weaker fixation, requiring a volar plaster splint. A clinical example is shown in Figure 3–12.

Distraction of the Wrist Joint Via a Triangular Fixation of the Radius to the First and Second Metacarpals

Yet another method distracts the wrist joint via a triangular fixation of the radius to the first and second metacarpals. Fixation is performed as for a standard distraction of the wrist joint with two accessory wires in the first metacarpal. The rods are connected in a triangular shape (Figure 3–13). The advantage of this method is that there can be simultaneous distraction of several articular fractures. A clinical example is shown in Figure 3–14.

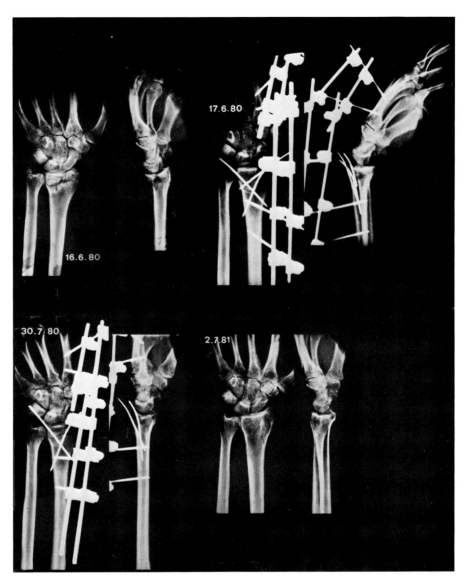

Figure 3–10 (cont.) B

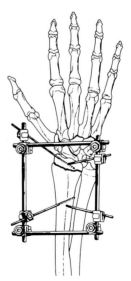

Figure 3–11 Frame fixation without crossing the wrist joint.

Wrist Fractures

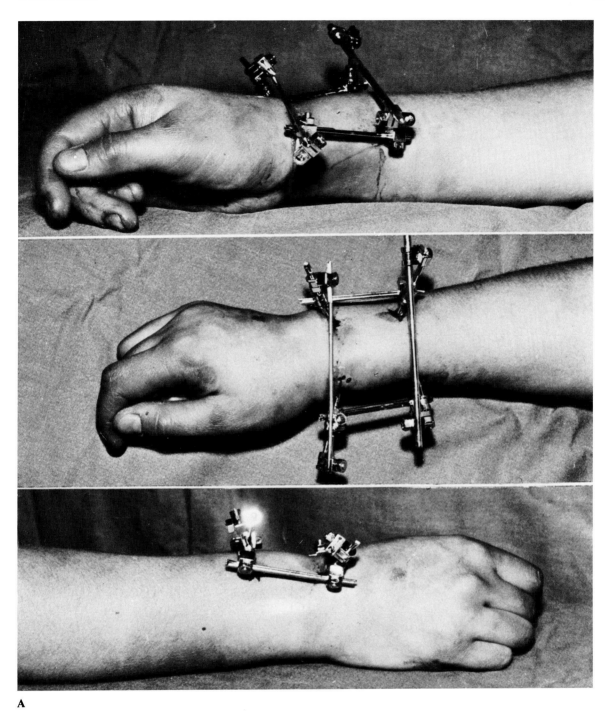

A

Figure 3–12 Dorsal tilt of a single distal radial fragment which could not be held reduced by flexion or by Kirschner wire fixation.

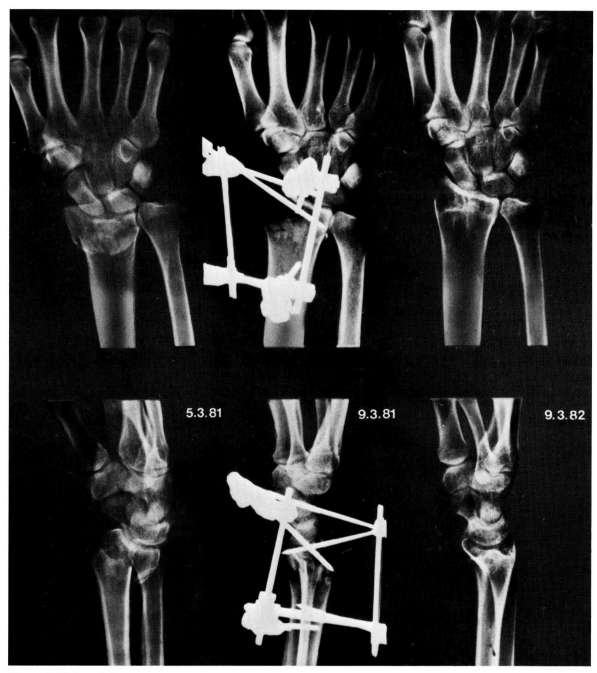

Figure 3–12 (cont.) B

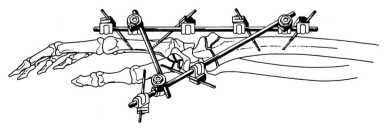

Figure 3–13 Distraction of the wrist joint using a triangular fixation of the radius to the first and second metacarpals.

Wrist Fractures

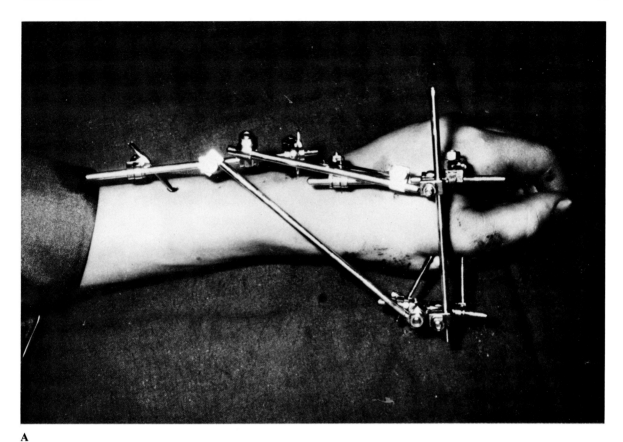

A

Figure 3–14 External fixator in a comminuted fracture of the distal radius and the base of the first metacarpal. Plate fixation of the distal ulna allows free rotation of the wrist joint.

Further Clinical Applications

Distraction of an Unstable Fracture of the Distal Radius in Combination With Internal Fixation of the Humerus, Radius, and Ulna

An unstable fracture of the distal radius can be distracted along with internal fixation of the humerus, radius, and ulna. The advantage to this procedure is that it facilitates soft tissue management and functional after-care. A clinical example is shown in Figure 3–15.

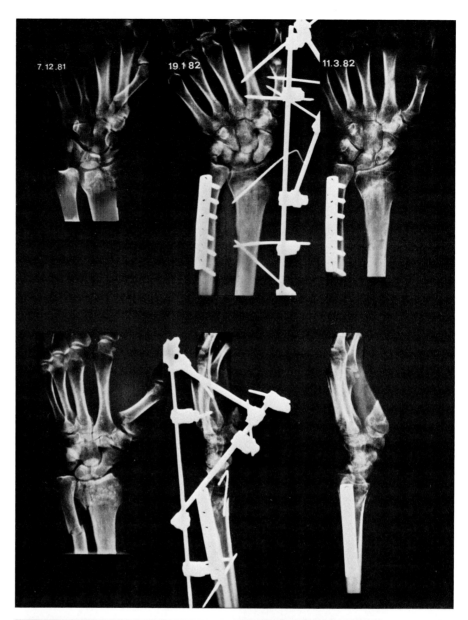

Figure 3–14 (cont.) B

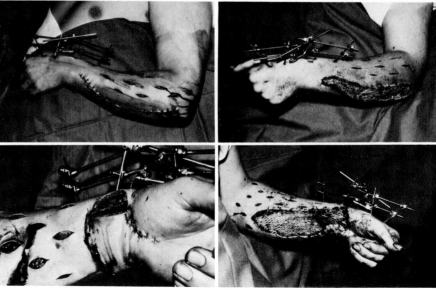

Figure 3–15 Crush injury of the left forearm with a comminuted fracture of the distal radius (extensor fixation) and proximal fracture of the forearm (plate fixation). Extensive dorsal and volar soft tissue release was required.

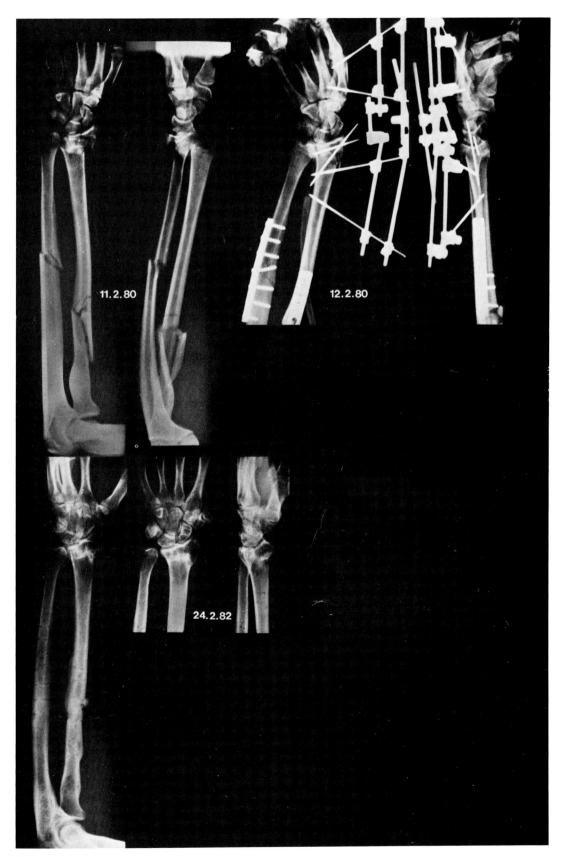

Figure 3–15 (cont.) B

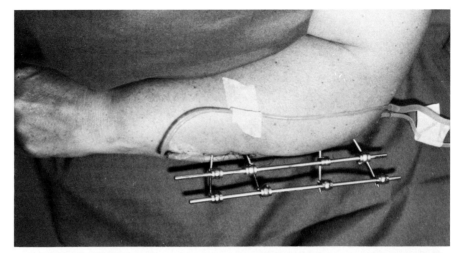
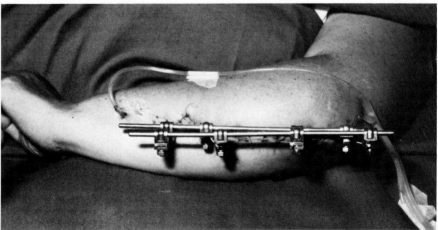

Figure 3-16 Infected plate osteosynthesis of the proximal ulna. Removal of the plate, debridement, resection of necrotic bone, suction drainage, and immobilization was accomplished in an external fixator; and a cancellous bone graft was applied after 3 weeks. Sufficient stability was provided by the external fixator to allow functional after-treatment and bony incorporation of the graft.

Osteitis of the Forearm

Osteitis of the forearm can be dealt with as shown in Figure 3-16.

Fracture Dislocation of the Foot

Fracture dislocation of the foot is illustrated in Figure 3-17.

Open Fractures in Small Children

Open fractures in small children may be treated as shown in Figure 3-18.

Wrist Fractures

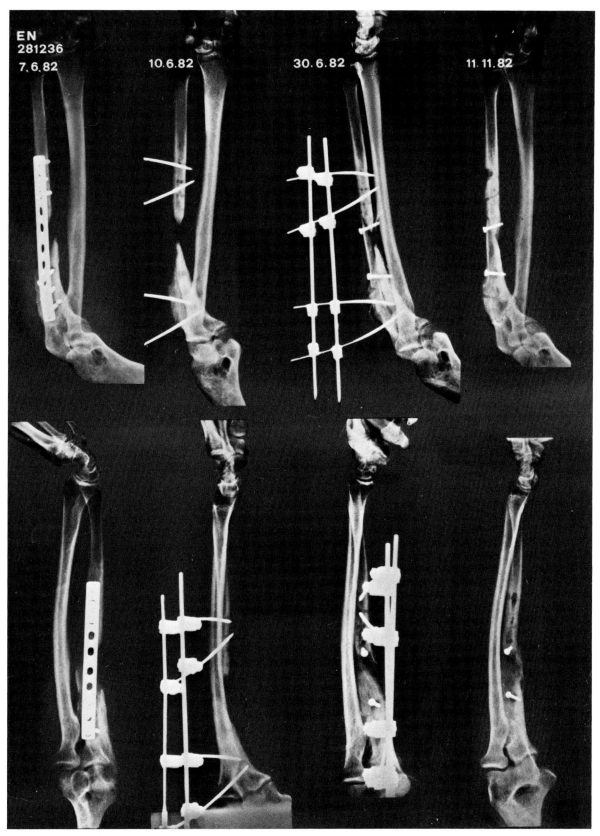

Figure 3–16 (cont.)

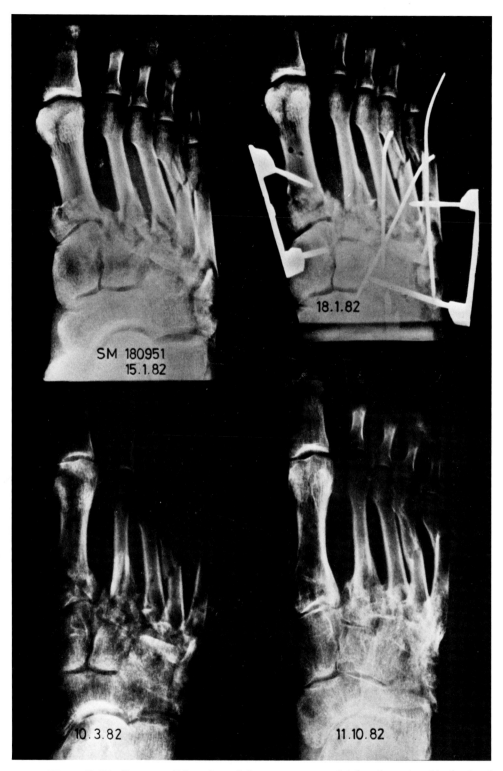

Figure 3–17 Fracture dislocation of the tarsometatarsal joint, 2 weeks old. A closed reduction was done, applying medial and lateral distraction. There was functional aftertreatment with concomitant pin fixation of the comminuted fractures of the os calcis. Consolidation occurred after 7 weeks.

Wrist Fractures

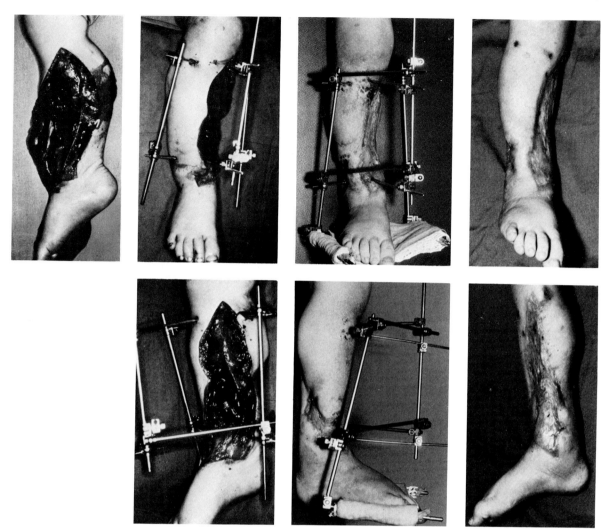

Figure 3–18 Third-degree open fracture of the lower leg with extensive segmental bone loss in an infant aged 20 months. Transfixation threaded pins were placed in the proximal and distal tibial metaphyses and were connected by the small fixator in a bilateral frame configuration. Stability was increased by triangulation with anterior threaded pins. A footplate was applied to prevent an equinus deformity. Mesh grafting of the skin was performed. After 10 weeks there was some spontaneous callus formation in the remaining periosteal tube. After 14 weeks there was interposition of a long cortical graft from the opposite tibia. The apparatus was removed after 20 weeks with the tibia united.

After-Treatment

A volar splint may be worn for four weeks for comfort, especially when only one rod is used. Radiologic assessment is recommended at 1, 2, 4, 7, and 8 weeks postoperatively. When reduction is being lost, distraction has to be increased. If distraction is applied in an extreme position of the wrist joint in order to maintain reduction, a neutral position must be regained after 2–3 weeks to minimize the risk of Sudeck's dystrophy.

In order to avoid pin tract infections, the edges of the skin around the pins must be without tension and are nursed daily. The pins are removed after 7–8 weeks. Physiotherapy is essential to maintain mobility of the finger and all other joints not immobilized by the external fixator.

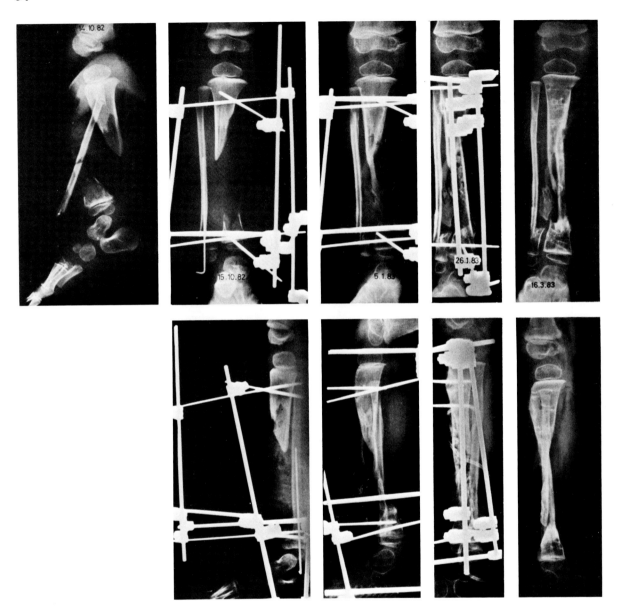

Figure 3–18 (cont.)

Complications

Complications are rare and are observed only in markedly unstable fractures. The following possible complications are listed according to their chronologic occurrence.

1. *Deviation of the pins during insertion.* Because of the risk of injury to the internal structures of the hand, the threaded pins must be inserted perpendicular to the cortex of the second metacarpal, thereby minimizing the risk of sliding off the bone.

Wrist Fractures

2. *Loss of reduction.* In unstable fractures frequent x-ray controls are necessary to detect loss of reduction. The distraction may have to be increased.
3. *Symptoms of median nerve impairment.* Disturbances of sensation in the distribution of the median nerve may be produced by too marked a distraction. The distraction may then have to be decreased.
4. *Pin tract infections.* The pin tracts must be nursed by the patient daily. The skin around the pins should be without any tension. If necessary, tight areas are released.
5. *Sudeck's dystrophy.* The incidence of this complication is low. It is mainly observed when the external fixator is applied late, i.e., 1–2 weeks after the fracture or when the wrist joint is fixed in an extreme position.
6. *Nonunion.* If a fracture extends into the metaphysis or diaphysis of the radius, decreased union of the fracture may be expected, especially with a patient older than 65 years. Further plaster fixation is then recommended, after removal of the fixator, for 3–5 weeks. If necessary, metaphyseal/diaphyseal plate fixation is useful.

Results

Since 1977 external fixation of the wrist joint has been used in over 100 patients. The comminuted fracture dislocation of the distal radius was by far the predominant indication. Application of this system was extended by hand surgeons.

Although a small number of the patients developed marked signs of osteoarthrosis, these were due to the severity of the intraarticular component of the fractures. The clinical results in regard to function, power, pain, and residual deformity of the wrist joint may be expected to be nearly always good or satisfactory. Our own experience (6,7) with 80% excellent and good results (including radiologic follow-up), is in accordance with the results of other authors (2–5,9).

Summary

The use of distraction in unstable fractures of the distal radius, the wrist joint, and the hand allows one to maintain an anatomic reduction until union of the fracture is achieved. It avoids circulatory disturbances by providing plaster-free after-treatment and allows unimpaired finger and elbow motion, thereby decreasing the risk of dystrophy. The hand is free for use in certain daily activities, which is an advantage, especially in patients with bilateral fractures.

Treatment with the external fixator is useful in the presence of a fracture of the distal radius in combination with multiple injuries of the upper extremity. This is true especially when extensive soft tissue injuries with vascular and/or neural involvement require an unimpaired approach for continued monitoring or management during the phase of after-treatment.

Acknowledgments

My thanks to M. E. Müller, R. Mathys, U. Büchler, D. Fernandez, P. Ballmer, and R. Ganz who have contributed to this technique and this work. Thanks also to J. Zysset for the drawings and D. Helfet for the critical reading of the English text.

REFERENCES

1. Anderson R, O'Neill G. (1944). Comminuted fractures of the end of the radius. Surg Gynecol Obstet 78:434.
2. Cooney WP (1978): Current management of fractures of the distal radius and forearm: experience with external pin fixation. In: External Fixation, The Current State of the Art, edited by Brooker AF, Edwards CC. Williams & Wilkins, Baltimore.
3. Cooney WP (1980). External mini-fixators: clinical applications and techniques. In: Advances in External Fixation, edited by Johnston RM. Year Book Publishers, Chicago.
4. Cooney WP, Linscheid RL, Dobyns JH (1979). External pin fixation for unstable Colles' fractures. J Bone Joint Surg 61A:840.
5. Grana WA, Kopta JA (1979). The Roger Anderson device in the treatment of fractures of the distal end of the radius. J Bone Joint Surg 61A:1234.
6. Jakob RP (1980): Die Distraktion instabiler distaler Radiustrümmerfrakturen mit einem Fixateur externe—ein neuer Behandlungsweg. Hefte Unfallheilk 148:99.
7. Jakob RP, Fernandez D (1982): The treatment of wrist fractures with the small AO fixation device. In: Current Concepts of External Fixation of Fractures. Springer-Verlag, Berlin.
8. Vidal J, Buscayret C, Connes H (1978): Treatment of articular fractures by "ligamento-taxis" with external fixation. In: External Fixation, the Current State of the Art, edited by Brooker AF, Edwards CC. Williams & Wilkins, Baltimore.

Stabilizing Hand Fractures with Tension Bands

4

Robert Belsole

Internal fixation of hand fractures is required when adequate reduction cannot be achieved or is lost subsequent to closed reduction and immobilization. Stabilization also is needed for displaced intraarticular fractures and when fractures are accompanied by significant injury to the soft tissue support systems, i.e., tendons, capsule, etc. Displaced fractures in the hand are stabilized to obtain reduction by overcoming deforming forces and to provide rigidity against redisplacement during postoperative mobilization. Fixed fractures are subjected to considerable forces when mobilizing the hand before sufficient callus forms. These stresses are greater than the initial deforming forces and should be the prime concern when planning and implementing fixation methods. Inadequately fixed fractures retard attempted movement of the digits and tend to displace. Although nonunion is rare, fractures that are insufficiently stabilized often heal with rotatory and/or angular malalignment. On the other hand, too much or "excessive" fixation increases the potential for severe joint contractures and tendon adhesions because of the increased surgical trauma that is frequently required.

Good hand function requires supple soft tissues, mobile joints, freely gliding tendons, adequate neural integrity, and an intact aligned skeleton. If one contemplates operative reduction, all requirements should be considered. Adequate fixation of fractures does not return the limb to optimal function unless its soft tissues are treated simultaneously. Fractures are stabilized to align the skeleton and allow early motion. Fixation should be sufficient to prevent redisplacement of fractured components during motion. A discussion of the minimal amount of fixation that achieves this goal is the purpose of this chapter.

Background

Many forms of internal fixation have been advanced for fractures of the hand. Wires, K-pins, compression screws, miniplates, and intramedullary pins have advantages in certain instances (3–6,9). Simple devices, e.g., wires and K-pins,

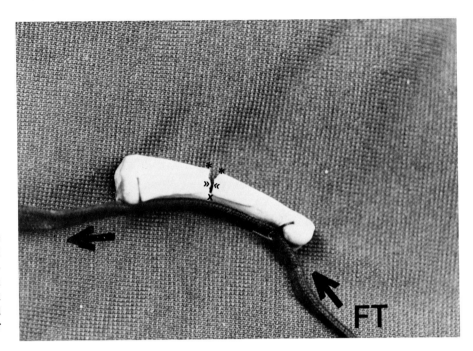

Figure 4-1 Transverse fractured phalangeal model under flexor tendon load. (**) tension cortex. (x) compression cortex. (≫≪) neutral bending axis. (*FT*) flexor tendon.

rely on ease of insertion and either cautious motion or complete immobilization. More refined engineering designs have made available devices for compression and/or rigid fixation that provide sufficient stabilization to allow early mobilization. These appliances and techniques, however, have increased dramatically in complexity. Most have been adopted from similar equipment/techniques used to treat fractures elsewhere in the body. More important than the equipment itself, however, has been the incorporation of mechanical principles that stress position of placement, efficacy of compression, and degrees of stability.

Tension Band Principle

The tension band principle was first introduced by Pauwels (7) and was applied to fracture surgery by Weber (10). A load generates tension and compression on opposing surfaces of a beam. On the tension side forces distract, whereas on the opposite side the load generates compression. If an external force or support is properly placed, it neutralizes tension that is generated by the load. Similarly, when loaded, a transverse fracture separates on the convex side and compresses on its concave surface (Figure 4-1). A tension band wire applied to the tension side of the same model neutralizes forces that tend to separate the fracture. Previously published reports demonstrated the use of tension band wires in transverse fractures and arthrodeses (1,9). A dorsally applied tension band wire neutralizes a load placed on the reduced fracture by the flexor tendon system. It should be emphasized that an arbitrary point exists in this fracture model equidistant between the dorsal and volar cortices at which neither tension or compression is generated (the neutral bending axis). Furthermore, although tension and compression is generated on either side of the axis during a load, both are maximal on opposing surfaces.

Tension and compression surfaces are less well defined in spiral and obliquely oriented fractures. Forces that tend to displace these fractures are multidirectional and influenced by fracture planes, tendon systems, and the

Stabilizing Hand Fractures

direction in which the load is applied. Tension bands can enhance stabilization by providing support against some, but not all, major displacing forces.

Experimental analyses of tension bands for fixation of small bones were undertaken using both standard biomechanical principles and a newly developed strain recording model (2,8). Only transverse osteotomies were studied because of simplicity and better control of experimental conditions. It was recognized that transversely oriented fractures are uncommon clinically.

Fifty-two fresh frozen pig metacarpals were osteotomized and mounted in epoxy. A transverse osteotomy was made in the midportion of the diaphysis. Experimental fractures were stabilized using dorsal figure-of-eight tension bands and three other common wiring techniques. Constructs were subjected to four-point bending on an Instron testing machine. Standard load deformation curves were produced as each specimen was tested to failure. Maximum peak load and deformation were plotted directly, and the stiffness (resistance of each stabilized construct to deformation) and the energy absorbed were measured directly from load deformation curves. The study concluded that figure-of-eight tension band fixation of transverse osteotomies provides high mechanical strength and excellent stiffness, and separates least when tested experimentally in four-point bending. Crossed K-wires provided suboptimal fixation when compared to other commonly employed fixation methods used in the study.

Because objective comparisons of various fixation techniques are difficult, we developed a strain recording model that eliminates biologic variations and produces sensitive measurements of fixation methods (Figure 4–2A). The experimental design allows evaluation of various forms of internal fixation in the same model by eliminating the necessity of testing constructs to the point of failure. Strain is the ratio of the change in length to the original length. When a fixed experimental construct is loaded in a cantilever system, the tensile cortex increases in length and produces positive strain (Figure 4–2B). If fixation is absent, no strain is observed. Likewise, compression or decreased length records a negative strain. Strain recordings of stabilized experimental transverse osteotomies reflect the strength of the fixation. The stronger the fixation, the greater is the magnitude of the strain recorded on either the tensile (+) or compressive (−) surfaces of the experimental model.

The study evaluated fixation of transverse osteotomies by wires placed on the dorsal cortex and through the neutral bending axis (Figure 4–2C,D). The results supported the tension band principle. Also, looped tension bands produced higher strain recordings than figure-of-eight bands, indicating that wire length and configuration are important considerations. Strain recordings also indicated that crossed K-wires alone provide less stability than techniques utilizing tension bands. Many questions remain unanswered, however, such as the effect of cyclic loading on all forms of fixation in the hand and the most advantageous wire gauge size, position, and tightening methods. Hopefully, strain recordings will facilitate investigations of these questions in the future.

Clinically, we have utilized modifications of tension band fixation in almost every type of acute fracture and corrective osteotomy of the hand. Techniques have been modified because of the wide spectrum of fractures that are usually encountered. The techniques are easily mastered but are not for the inexperienced surgeon. The incorporation of these methods into one's surgical armamentarium requires a sufficient knowledge of operative stabilization techniques that facilitate dextrous tasks, e.g., drilling small holes through fracture fragments sometimes at rather unusual angles, placing small K-pins, and passing and tightening stainless steel wires. Proper handling of soft tissues is obligatory. Techniques are discussed below based on specific types of fractures. K-wires are referred to as K-pins to avoid confusion with stainless steel wires.

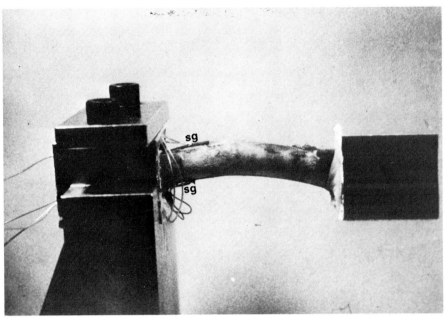

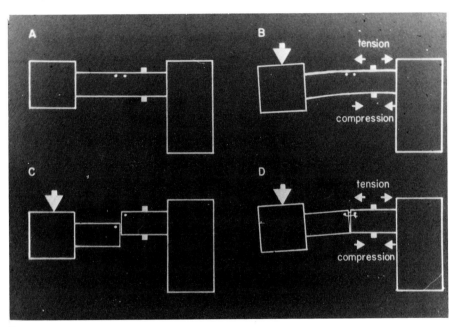

Figure 4–2 Strain comparisons of tension band wiring of experimental transverse fractures. **A** Cantilever-system-mounted specimen in epoxy with strain gauges (*sg*) attached. **B** Strain measurement hypothesis. *A, B:* An intact bone generates tension and compression when loaded. The increase and decrease in length is recorded as strain. *C:* When osteotomized and loaded without fixation, no strain is recorded. *D:* Fixed construct allows strain to be generated. The stronger the fixation, the higher the strain recorded. Stabilizing methods can be compared in the same model if application of the load remains constant.

Stabilizing Hand Fractures

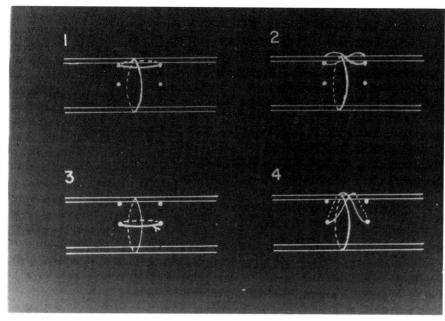

C

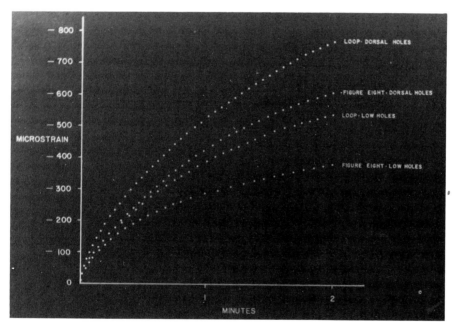

D

Figure 4–2 (cont.) C Comparison of wire fixations placed through the dorsal cortex and neutral bending axis. Loop and figure-of-eight configurations are also compared. **D** Graph illustrating strain recordings of fractures stabilized (C1–C4) and subjected to cantilever bending.

Techniques

Because of its vital importance, postoperative management is discussed before the surgical techniques. When needed, operative stabilization of fractures in the hand initiates, rather than concludes, the treatment. A strict postoperative protocol is followed. For 3–5 days after surgery, the hand and wrist are immobi-

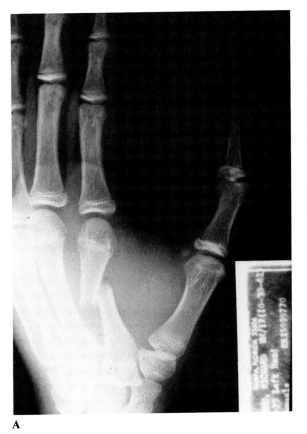

Figure 4–3 Transverse fracture. **A** Transverse fracture of the index metacarpal. The initial reduction was lost at 3 days during immobilization. **B,C** Intraoperative photographs demonstrating tension band wiring. Note the 18-gauge needle that is used to protect tissues during the drilling of transverse holes. In this case, a double loop tightening was utilized. **D** Roentgenogram showing postoperative reduction.

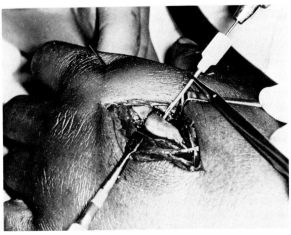

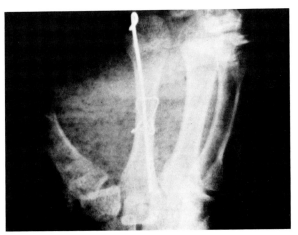

lized in the position of best "ultimate function." Volar and dorsal plasters position the wrist at 40° extension, the metacarpophalangeal (MCP) joints in 70°–90° of flexion, and the interphalangeal (IP) joints in 0°–10° of flexion. The thumb remains free unless the first ray is injured, at which time it is maintained in full abduction and extension. After 3 days the dressings and splint are removed and the wounds assessed. The wrist *only* is splinted in extension for 3 weeks, during which time active mobilization of the digits and thumb is started. Pinch is discouraged. At 3 weeks the splint is removed and formal hand therapy initiated if needed. Lifting heavy objects is not allowed for 6 weeks. Dynamic extension splints are applied if required.

Stabilizing Hand Fractures

Surgical Technique—General

All open reductions and fixations are performed under axillary or general anesthesia. Tourniquets are applied to the upper brachium and inflated to 80 mm Hg above the systolic blood pressure. Using loupe magnification, fractures are approached dorsally through slightly curved incisions unless wounds exist that require meticulous debridement during entry. Metacarpals are approached on either side of the extensor tendons. Junctura tendinia are preserved. If needed for exposure, they are divided, marked, and later repaired. When exposing phalangeal fractures, either the extensor mechanism is divided in the midplane or the fracture rent is enlarged proximally and distally. Periosteal tissues are elevated to allow identification of the fractured fragments. Complete visualization of the injury is imperative. Fractures are reduced and held with bone-holding forceps. When multiple fragments are encountered, two major elements are reduced, held, and stabilized, after which other components are affixed to the major unit. Intraarticular fractures are reduced and stabilized under direct vision of cartilage surfaces. After tension bands are applied, all tissues are returned to their original anatomic continuum, including lacerated nerves and tendons. If there is significant soft tissue injury, the postoperative protocol is adjusted accordingly. K-pins of 0.062 inch (1.6 mm), 0.045 inch (1.1 mm), 0.035 inch (0.89 mm), and 0.028 inch (0.71 mm) are drilled with power. Stainless steel surgical wires, 26 gauge (0.4 mm; No. 0) or 24 gauge (0.51 mm; No. 2), are passed around K-pins or through holes drilled with a 0.035-inch K-pin. K-pins are usually left beneath the skin and later removed in the office if they produce symptoms. Surgical wires are tightened by hand with a needle-holder and cut off, and then the twisted ends are placed flat on the bone.

Transversely Oriented Fractures

Metacarpal Fractures

Transverse metacarpal fractures can be unstable especially if interlocking surfaces are absent (Figures 4–3A–D). The cross section of metacarpal midshafts are unusually small, making crossed K-pinning difficult. These fractures can be fixed with larger longitudinal K-pins (0.062 and 0.045 inch) that are drilled distally from the fracture surface to exit beneath the collateral ligaments. After reduction, the pin is drilled retrogradely across the fracture site. Positioning the pin under the collateral ligament allows full MCP motion. A dorsal tension band wire (24 or 26 gauge) is passed through two drill holes placed parallel and equidistant from the fracture. A figure-of-eight or loop configuration of the wire may be used. We now favor a simple loop that is singly tied. The holes that house the tension wires should be dorsal to the neutral bending axis and as close to the cortex as possible. The K-pin is left externally and removed in 4–6 weeks.

Phalangeal Fractures

Transverse fractures and osteotomies are very difficult to secure. Small, flat, opposing surfaces minimize good surface apposition. Adequate reduction is difficult to judge, and small discrepancies of alignment produce rather severe malunions that decrease function. Hyperextension deformities are common and are compensated by distal flexion contractures. X-ray control is suggested. Med-

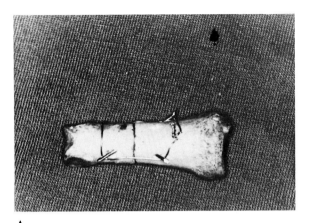 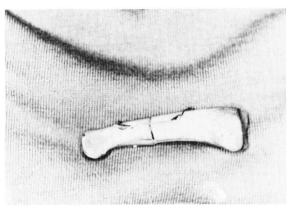

Figure 4–4A,B Fractured proximal phalangeal model stabilized with dorsal K-pins and a tension band wire.

ullary pins can be placed to obtain longitudinal alignment. These pins are removed after dorsal tension banding is accomplished. Two crossed K-pins are drilled dorsal to the neutral axis (Figure 4–4A,B). The pins in this position also counteract the separation of the dorsal cortex. A stainless steel wire (26 or 28 gauge) incorporates the proximal and distal protuding pins. Exactly reduced fractures can also be stabilized with a diagonal K-pin and a dorsal tension band wire placed in a fashion similar to that described for metacarpal fractures. This is not suggested for osteotomies because correction may be lost when the wire is tightened. Transverse fractures of the middle phalanx are best handled by a longitudinal K-pin that transfixes the fracture and the distal interphalangeal joint and exits under the nail. This is supplemented by a dorsal tension wire through bone on either side of the fracture.

Long Spiral Oblique Fractures

Metacarpal Fractures

After reduction, long oblique metacarpal fractures are secured by one or more combinations of K-pins and wires. When involved, joint surfaces are aligned first with K-pins. Additional pins are drilled through major fracture components. Properly placed K-pins avoid fracture lines and lie in a plane almost perpendicular to the fracture. Two major fractured components can be stabilized by two K-pins that are placed a considerable distance apart from each other so long as each pin penetrates good bone and avoids fracture interfaces (Figures 4–5A,B). If the bone is visualized as a cylinder, the pins are made to enter and exit each component at angles that allow the stainless steel wire to incorporate the greatest circumference. The wire envelops the ends of the protruding K-pins and spans the fracture, compressing and exerting its tension band effect against the major displacing force—rotation of the distal component.

Phalangeal Fractures

Most long oblique phalangeal fractures involve articular surfaces and possess less spiral configuration than do the metacarpal injuries. The bone is relatively uniform in shape and is flattened rather than rounded in its midportion.

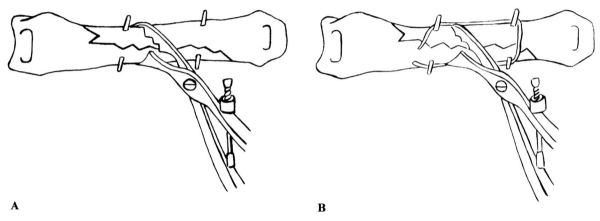

Figure 4–5A,B Fixation technique applied to a long spiral oblique fracture of the metacarpal. Banding wire envelops protruding k-pins and are placed without removing the bone clamp. Wires are cut off, tied, and laid flat on bone (not shown).

Techniques are similar to metacarpal fixation except smaller pins and wires are employed (0.028 or 0.035 inch; 26 or 28 gauge, respectively). Joint surfaces are restored initially and anatomically. Wires are passed dorsally across the surface of the bone and, if required, placed volarly. If one is concerned about violating the flexor tendon sheath, volar wires may be passed through small drill holes in the volar cortex.

Short Spiral Oblique Fractures

Metacarpal/Phalangeal Fractures

Short oblique fractures are troublesome because of the limited amount of fracture surfaces. When loaded, the shear forces are greater. Additional pins are required, with their planes of insertion lying directly perpendicular to the bone and to the fracture. When the fracture includes cartilage, we prefer to insert one pin at right angles to the bone to reduce the joint, and one or more pins perpendicular to the fracture plane for compression (Figures 4–6A–D). Both K-pins can be enveloped individually with small tension wires. These wires also serve to anchor sutures needed to repair the capsule and ligaments.

Complex Fractures

Metacarpal/Phalangeal Fractures

Wire/K-pin combinations are contraindicated in injuries with extensive comminution or bone loss. When coapting fracture surfaces are absent, tension band wires are unable to exert sufficient force against displacement. Frequently the fracture collapses, especially if motion is attempted.

However, many fractures can be secured by modifying the technique and rebuilding the bone unit in stages (Figures 4–7A–C). Operative planning is crucial, and bands are placed in as many planes as possible to counteract multidirectional forces. Volarly passed wires that encircle K-pins placed at reverse angles enhance stability between individually fixed components.

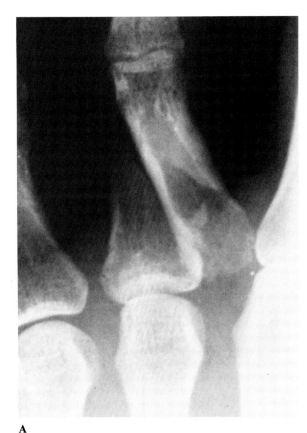

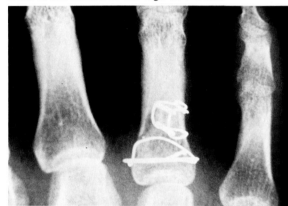

Figure 4–6 Short spiral oblique fracture stabilized with the author's technique. **A–C** Fracture fixation. **D** There is full flexion of the digit at 6 weeks.

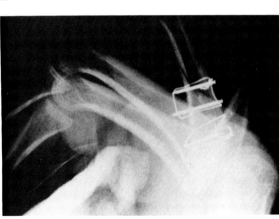

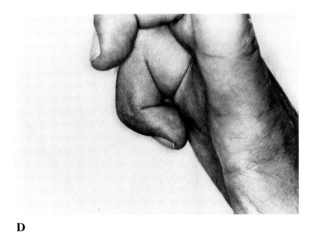

Summary

Tension band wiring provides a good alternative when stabilizing hand fractures. In many instances, wire/K-pin combinations alleviate the need for plate application on small bones. The technique and its modifications stress position in regard to potential displacement under the load produced by early motion. Experimental studies are being directed toward discovery of the actual amount of fixation required. Smaller caliber wires and pins as well as newer carbide and synthetic materials may someday further reduce the amount of materials needed to physiologically stabilize these injuries.

Stabilizing Hand Fractures

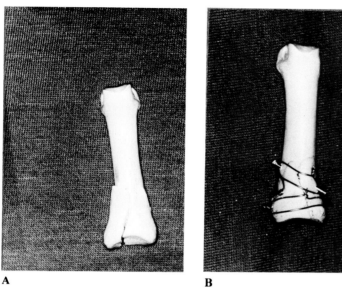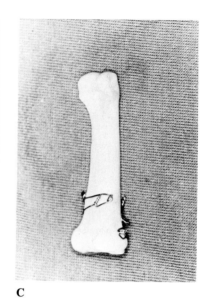

A   **B**   **C**

Figure 4–7 This three-part phalangeal fracture illustrates the modified tension band technique. **A** Intraarticular fracture. **B,C** The joint is first reduced, after which proximal and distal components are united and stabilized with dorsal (**B**) and volar (**C**) K-pin wire configurations.

REFERENCES

1. Allende BT, Engelem JC (1980). Tension band arthrodeses in the finger joints. J Hand Surg 5:269.
2. Gould WL, Rayhack J, Belsole RJ, Skelton, WH (1984). Tension band stabilization of transverse fractures: an experimental analysis. Plast Reconstr Surg (in press).
3. Green DP, Anderson JR (1973). Closed reduction and percutaneous pin fixation of fractured phalanges. J Bone Joint Surg 55A:1651.
4. Heim V (1974). Small Fragment Set Manual. Springer-Verlag, New York.
5. Kilbourne BC, Paul EG (1958). The use of small bone screws in the treatment of metacarpal, metatarsal and phalangeal fractures. J Bone Joint Surg 40A:375.
6. Lister G (1978). Intraosseous wiring of the digital skeleton. J Hand Surg 3:427.
7. Pauwels F (1935). Der Schenkelhalsbruch Ein Metanisches. Problem Enke, Stuttgart.
8. Rayhack JM, Belsole RJ, Skelton WH (1984). A strain recording model: analysis of fracture fixation in small bones. J Hand Surg (in press).
9. Segmuller G (1977). Surgical Stabilization of the Skeleton of the Hand. Williams & Wilkins, Baltimore.
10. Weber BK (1963). Grundlagen und Maglich Keiten der Zuggurtungsosteosynthese. Chirurg 35:81–86.

Multiple Trauma and Pelvic Bleeding: Diagnosis and Treatment

5

R. Y. McMurtry

The majority of pelvic fractures pose neither a diagnostic nor a therapeutic problem. They occur in an older population, typically postmenopausal females, and follow a relatively low-energy injury. Generally on x-ray a relatively undisplaced anterior fracture is noted involving the superior or inferior ramus. Even though studies (2) have shown that there is commonly posterior involvement on a bone scan, the patient's management is straightforward. Treatment is essentially symptomatic; that is, the patient may ambulate as comfort permits. Given present health cost restraints, the majority of these patients are being treated on an outpatient basis. Indeed, it is of interest how well outpatient management of these injuries is succeeding in our center.

This type of pelvic injury, however, is not the focus of this chapter. Rather, a more serious pelvic injury is associated with a younger age group and high-energy type injuries. In previous publications (6,8), we identified a 20% incidence of pelvic fractures in the multiply injured patient. This percentage has remained constant over more than 7 years of experience with 1,500 patients. In contrast to the first group of pelvic fractures, these injuries present a significant therapeutic problem. Not all of these fractures are intrinsically life-threatening, but they do indicate the degree of energy transfer that occurred during the actual injury. The types of pelvic fractures that are of concern in terms of morbidity and mortality are the "posterior" or unstable pelvic fractures (3,5,8), open fractures, and fractures associated with major vessel injury. In all of the foregoing groups, mortality rates of up to 50% have been identified. The purpose of this chapter is to review a consecutive series of 109 multiply injured patients with these problem pelvic fractures, highlighting the management of associated bleeding and appropriate treatment methods.

Review of 109 Pelvic Fractures

We have conducted a review (7) of 109 patients who had pelvic fractures and other injuries. As has been the case since our trauma unit opened, all patients have been prospectively documented as to their age, sex, mechanism of injury, injury severity score (ISS), vital signs, hematology, coagulogram (platelet count, partial thromboplastin time, and prothrombin time), blood gases, the injury sustained, and operations carried out. From April 1981 to December 1982 inclusively, there were 487 patients treated in the trauma unit, of whom 109 sustained pelvic fractures. There were 63 males and 46 females with an 18% mortality rate (19 patients). The average patient age was 34 (range 14–87), and the average ISS was 31 (range 16–75). Of the 19 who died, there were 10 males and nine females with an average age of 45 and an average ISS of 46 for all ages and an ISS of 53 for those under 50 years of age. Hemorrhage was present in 19 of these mortalities and unstable pelvic fractures in 11.

For the purposes of this chapter, it is pertinent to focus on three aspects of the problem: mortality, unstable pelvic fractures, and bleeding. Shock was considered to be present if the systolic blood pressure was beneath 90 mm Hg and/or the pulse rate was over 120/min. Hemorrhage was deemed to have occurred if greater than one blood volume of replacement blood was required. Unstable pelvic fractures were defined if the sacroiliac complex was completely disrupted, i.e., through the sacrum, ilium, or the sacroiliac joint (including the posterior sacroiliac ligaments). This determination was made on the basis of review of anteroposterior, inlet, and outlet views of the pelvis.

Given these definitions, there is an obvious relationship between shock and unstable pelvic fractures because 38 (62%) of the shocked patients had disruption of their sacroiliac complex. By contrast, only 24 (34%) of the 70 patients with stable pelvic fractures were in shock. When other injuries are taken into account, however, the number of true pelvic bleeds is of interest. Only 21 cases were calculated to have lost one blood volume or more solely from pelvic causes. Of these, 17 (81%) had unstable fractures. There were seven deaths among these 21 cases (33%) six of which were in patients with unstable fractures.

The most important finding in this review, however, was that of coagulopathy. Fourteen patients were noted to have a partial thromboplastin time at least 1.5 times normal during initial resuscitation; of these patients, 12 (86%) died. The average number of transfusions given to these patients averaged 47 units (range 5–97). Clearly, coagulopathy is a very bad prognostic sign.

Based on this review, unstable pelvic fractures are prone to be associated with more injuries, bleeding, and a higher mortality rate (Table 5–1). If a coagulopathy develops, survival becomes unlikely. When discussing management therefore, it is appropriate to focus on these high-risk cases.

Table 5–1. Unstable vs. Stable Pelvic Fractures

Parameter	No. of patients	
	Stable	Unstable
Total	70	39
Shock	24	38
Mortalities	8	11
Injury severity score (average)	27	35
Pelvic Bleeds	4	17
Coagulopathy	1	13

Management

In general, rapid resuscitation and control of bleeding accomplished within a minimal time frame is the desired goal of care in these patients. The difficulty that arises with most pelvic fractures is management of the associated hemorrhage. The bleeding may be from the pelvis itself, associated injuries, or both. The difficulty arises in the immediate identification of the source(s) of blood loss.

The three major possibilities of blood loss in blunt trauma are thoracic and intra- and extraperitoneal injuries. The first (thoracic) is readily appreciated by chest x-ray and chest tube insertion. Excessive drainage of blood is readily quantified and thoracotomy pursued for surgical control. The intra- and extraperitoneal components, however, are more difficult diagnostic problems. Although minilaparotomy is very useful in patients with blunt trauma, its usefulness after pelvic fractures is limited owing to a 15% false-positive rate in our experience—even with the supraumbilical approach. If negative, however, the problem becomes simplified, and all therapeutic efforts may then focus on the problem of the pelvic fracture. If the minilaparotomy is positive, one must assume that there are at least two sources of bleeding to be managed. Additionally, administering 7–8 units of platelets and 3 units of fresh frozen plasma for each 5 liters of intravenous replacement is very useful. With this protocol our survival rate of patients receiving 20 units or more of blood during the first 24 hr has risen to over 50%.

Specific Management

The most important component in specific management is early recognition of the patient at risk. The problems with pelvic hemorrhage are most likely to develop under two circumstances: a major vessel injury or loss of tamponade. Major vessel injury occurred in less than 5% of the 188 cases we have reviewed to date (6,7). What is far more frequent is the loss of tamponade, which occurs from two sources: One is the unstable pelvic fracture with significant displacement, and the other is the open pelvic fracture. In the former, the displaced pelvis allows expansion of the extraperitoneal space to two to three times its normal volume, which means that far more blood is lost before tamponade occurs. With open fractures, once there is communication with the environment, tamponade does not occur and there is a corresponding increased risk of significant hemorrhage. Clearly then, management must be geared to anticipate these particular problems. As indicated in Table 5–2, there are four specific measures that may be used: pneumatic shock garment, reduction of the fracture, surgery, and angiography.

Pneumatic Antishock Garment

The principle role of the pneumatic antishock garment is as a first-aid measure and for patient transfer. Its use has also been described (1) after other definitive surgical management, but we have no experience with that aspect and indeed do not recommend it. The advantages of the pneumatic antishock garment are that it is quick, simple, and safe and has the potential of three beneficial effects: hemostasis, autotransfusion, and increased peripheral vascular resistance. This in turn results in decreased ongoing blood loss, a measurable increase in venous return and central venous pressure, and finally a significant improvement in mean arterial pressure.

The disadvantages of the garment, however, are significant. The principle one is the loss of access to and visibility of the abdomen and lower extremities. It literally renders impossible meaningful clinical assessment of these areas. Although x-ray films can be obtained through the garment, little other information can be gained. The advent of the transparent pneumatic antishock garment helps in this respect, but it does not solve all the problems. The garment also eliminates access to the abdomen and lower extermities for therapeutic interventions, e.g., groin cutdowns.

In our own institution, we feel that every effort should be made to remove the pneumatic antishock garment at the earliest opportunity. If the patient becomes unstable during the release, however, removal should be carried out only in the operating room. This subject is more completely discussed in the article by Pelligra and Sandberg (9).

Reduction of the Fracture

Reduction of the fracture represents the single most important step that can be taken for pelvic fractures associated with loss of tamponade effect. Because the most common cause of loss of tamponade is the displaced pelvis, the techniques that are available for reduction of the pelvis should be familiar to all orthopaedists who manage trauma. They are:

1. Anterior external fixation
2. Spica cast
3. Traction
4. Internal fixation

Of the foregoing, the most practical is the anterior external fixation device. A patient lying on the operating table undergoing laparotomy with the pelvis splayed open is virtually guaranteed ongoing and significant bleeding. In these cases it is imperative that the pelvis be reduced. This poses a significant dilemma because often the general surgeons are dealing with a significant source of bleeding elsewhere. Clearly, priority must be given to the source of bleeding associated with the greatest loss, but the decision as to which lesion that is can challenge the wisdom of Solomon. With expertise, reduction of the pelvic fracture by an anterior external frame can be accomplished within 15–20 min. Because this is by far the most rapid of the two maneuvers (i.e., compared to laparotomy), it is the one that should be accomplished first. This does not solve all the problems, however, because the frame itself may get in the way of the general surgeon, also an unacceptable problem. In our view, there is a need to design a simple device that can function as a temporary reduction clamp for the pelvis that may be applied in 3–5 min and that does not in any way interfere with a laparotomy. This is technically feasible, and we anticipate reporting on it in future communications.

The point is reemphasized that a displaced and unstable pelvic fracture must be viewed as a life-threatening injury. Reduction must be achieved at the earliest opportunity by the simplest available means. Indeed, it may not be possible to *await* cardiopulmonary stability because the reduction of the fracture may be the major means of overcoming ongoing bleeding.

We have little experience in the use of the other reduction modalities (i.e., spica cast and internal fixation) in the acute situation. The spica cast has

Multiple Trauma/Pelvic Bleeding

been used elsewhere (4) with reports of very good success. In the absence of expertise with the application of external fixation, a spica cast is recommended as a second line of defense. We likewise view traction as a method of reduction that is to be used as a back-up if other, more definitive means cannot be used.

Finally, our use of internal fixation is confined to very unstable pelvic fractures associated with complete sacroiliac disruption. On these occasions it is necessary to accomplish an open reduction and internal fixation of the sacroiliac joint. Unfortunately, this intervention is associated with significant blood loss and is of itself a challenge to a patient and quite possibly one they cannot stand in the early hours. For this reason, it is something that we tend to defer until the patient has been stabilized hemodynamically for 24–48 hr. Once internal fixation has been accomplished, however, it is very striking as to how stable the pelvis becomes and indeed how comfortable the patient is.

Surgical Control

Direct surgical management of pelvic fractures is indicated under three circumstances: (a) open fractures; (b) major vessel injury; and (c) patient in extremis.

Open Fractures

With open fractures, the necessity for surgery is that which exists for any open fracture. Specifically, appropriate debridement needs to be accomplished and all contaminated material removed. Management of the pelvic fracture should proceed along the lines described previously, preferably with an external fixation device. If supplementary internal fixation is required, particularly for the posterior sacroiliac joint, it should be carried out when cardiopulmonary stability has been achieved.

Major Vessel Injury

In our own experience, major vessel injury associated with blunt pelvic trauma is relatively uncommon, occurring in less than 5% of patients (i.e., seven of 188). Most of those patients have presented in extremis and therefore demanded surgical control, as is outlined subsequently. Major vessels cannot be controlled by angiography, and indeed the time spent with angiography is probably ill-advised because early surgical control is obligatory if survival is to be achieved.

Patient In Extremis

When a patient presents in severe shock after blunt trauma, it is necessary to follow a "crash protocol." The protocol used at our institution is outlined in Table 5–2. If the patient remains in shock in spite of the measures indicated in the protocol, direct surgical intervention is required. Specifically, the distal aorta is reached via a transperitoneal approach and is temporarily clamped. As swiftly as possible, the bleeding must be identified more distally so that the aortic clamp can be removed. The clamp should be applied as closely as possible to the bifurcation and left on for a maximum of 20 min, preferably less. Selective clamping of the major bleeding may then be carried out and "catch-up" replacement done. If the source of bleeding is not obvious, the pelvis should be packed so as to permit release of the aortic clamp. All major vessels

Table 5–2. Crash Protocol

Crash protocol should be instituted when a patient is in stage IV shock (American College of Surgeons' definition) or likely to be. The decision is to be made by the trauma team leader or the on-duty emergency physician. The following steps must be taken:

1. Call the trauma team.
2. Call the chief surgical resident who is to be part of the trauma team.
3. Notify the general surgical and anesthesia staff member that the "crash protocol" is in effect.
4. Notify the operating room the "crash protocol" is in effect.
5. Implement the following therapeutic interventions upon a patient's arrival:
   a. Endotracheal intubation.
   b. Bilateral chest tubes.
   c. Two or more large-bore IVs, No. 14 in diameter or larger, utilizing a bilateral groin cutdown if necessary.
   d. Apply the pneumatic antishock garment.
   e. Give 1–1.5 units blood volume replacement.
   f. Transfer to the operating room if there is a failure to respond once these measures are complete.

The above measures should be accomplished in 10–15 min.

should be checked; that is, the common, internal, and external iliac and femoral arteries and veins must be inspected. Any damage to them must be repaired in the usual fashion. If no obvious source of bleeding is found among these vessels, one must assume that the bleeding is from the internal iliac system and should proceed to the next diagnostic therapeutic option of angiography. However, it must be emphasized that prior to undertaking angiography reduction of the pelvic fracture should be accomplished by the most expeditious means possible because in most instances that maneuver is sufficient to deal with the bleeding in the small-bore vessels.

Angiography

Having had the experience of 3–4 years of angiography, we have concluded that its role is secondary to the foregoing measures. Its particular usefulness is in ongoing pelvic bleeding if the bleeding continues after the above measures have been accomplished: Specifically, all intraperitoneal bleeding has been dealt with, major vessel injury has either been ruled out or repaired, and the pelvic fracture has been reduced. Yet, if in spite of these measures the patient has ongoing bleeding and if coagulopathy has been excluded, angiography becomes warranted. The first step is to perform a pelvic aortogram, thus gaining some knowledge of the major arterial anatomy. This may or may not give the location of the bleeding site. More frequently, selective internal iliac arteriography is required. This permits more precise localization of the bleeding sites; which are identified by focal extravasation of contrast material in the arterial phase which often persists well into the capillary and venous phases. In addition to extravasation, there may be focal spasm and displacement or compression of vessels due to hematoma as indicators of the bleeding.

Once the bleeders are identified, therapeutic angiography may be considered. This may involve the use of autologous blood (25 cc) which is allowed to clot. If there is some problem with coagulopathy, fragments of gel foam can be used instead. The disadvantage of gel foam, however, is that it tends to produce permanent occlusion of the arteries and thus inadvertent embolization of important nonbleeding arteries, which could have serious consequences.

Multiple Trauma/Pelvic Bleeding

After selection of the embolic material, the bleeding sites are then selectively embolized under radiologic control until it is believed that no further extravasation is present.

Summary

Unstable pelvic fractures continue to be associated with significant morbidity and mortality. A treatment plan that emphasizes good general resuscitation while focusing on immediate reduction of the unstable pelvis is likely to achieve improved results in most of these difficult cases.

REFERENCES

1. Batalden DJ, Wickstrom PH, Ruiz E (1974). Value of G-suit in patients with severe pelvic fracture. Arch Surg 109:708–713.
2. Gertzbein SD, Chenoweth DR (1977). Occult injuries of the pelvic ring. Clin Orthop 128:202.
3. Gilliland MD, Ward RE, Barton RM (1982). Factors affecting mortality in pelvic fractures. J Trauma 22:691–693.
4. Hansen ST (1983). Personal communication.
5. Loosner KG, Crombie HD Jr (1976). Pelvic fractures: an anatomic guide to severity of injury. Am J Surg 132:638.
6. McMurtry RY (1983). General assessment and management of the polytraumatized patient. Cited by Tile M (ed.): Fractures of the Pelvis and Acetabulum. Williams & Wilkins, Baltimore.
7. McMurtry RY, Joyce M, et al. (1984). Pelvic fractures and bleeding: a review of 109 cases of polytraumatized patients. (in press).
8. McMurtry RY, Walton D, Dickinson D, et al. (1980). Pelvic disruption in the polytraumatized patient: a management protocol. Clin Orthop 151:22–30.
9. Pelligra R, Sandberg ED (1979). Control of intractable abdominal bleeding by external counter pressure JAMA 241:708–713.

Ender Nailing of Intertrochanteric Fractures of the Femur

6

James P. Waddell

Most surgeons accept that surgical treatment of trochanteric fractures of the femur in the elderly yields results superior to those of nonoperative treatment. Since the introduction of Smith-Peterson's first internal fixation device for fractures of the femoral neck, various devices have been designed or advocated for fixation of fractures of the intertrochanteric region.

The goal of operative treatment of trochanteric fractures is early weight-bearing stability using simple and nonradical surgical techniques. It is well recognized that prolonged recumbency is poorly tolerated by the elderly, and therefore any method of treatment which allows early ambulation with weight-bearing is desirable.

The surgical treatment of stable fractures of the intertrochanteric region does not present any particular problem aside from the morbidity and mortality seen with fractures of the elderly. Because of the inherent stability of the fracture, special demands for secure fixation are not encountered.

The loss of medial and posterior support in comminuted and displaced intertrochanteric fractures results in the loss of inherent stability. Because there is no capacity for the medial or compression side of the femur to absorb weight-bearing stresses (5,37,39), all of the force during ambulation must be absorbed by the fixation device. Therefore the goal of operative treatment which allows early ambulation and weight-bearing is much more difficult to achieve in unstable than in stable fractures.

This goal has been pursued via three paths. The first path was that of finding a stronger device. It was recognized that with many two-piece devices (e.g., the Thornton nail and McLaughlin side plate) and some one-piece devices (e.g., the Neufeld nail and the Moe plate) that insufficient strength in the implant was present to prevent bending and breaking of the implant with weight-bearing. Therefore devices such as the Holt nail (14) and the Sarmiento nail (35) were designed to permit the normal stresses of weight-bearing to be absorbed by

77

the fixation device without failure of the device. Because of the osteoporotic nature of the bone, however, protrusion of the nail in unstable fractures frequently occurred (7).

The second path followed in the search of fracture stability was a surgical modification of the fracture to convert an unstable fracture to a stable fracture and thus allow weight-bearing without undue stress being placed on the fixation device. Dimon and Hughston (7) described the medial displacement osteotomy, and Sarmiento (36) reported on a modification of this osteotomy with greater emphasis on valgus orientation of the proximal fragment and without medial displacement of the distal fragment. By rendering these fractures stable, the bones themselves were forced to share some of the stresses crossing the fracture site, thus protecting the implant from premature fatigue or failure. Such surgical modification may result in excessive shortening of the limb, malrotation, and late valgus deformity of the knee (33). Additionally, the magnitude of the surgery increases morbidity and mortality (16).

The third path followed in this search for stability involved the use of various sliding screws and nails. First described by Pohl in 1956 (38), the concept of a sliding screw within a cannulated firmly fixed side plate has become very attractive and is the base design for a number of similar devices currently available for use (28). The concept is essentially one of an intramedullary device which allows impaction of the fracture with weight-bearing while maintaining proper rotational orientation and preventing varus deformity through the fracture site. Failure of the device to slide results in complications similar to those seen with fixed devices (25).

Of the three paths chosen in the search for fracture stability, probably the concept of the sliding intramedullary device is the most widely accepted and used (8). This concept is often combined with the first two, however, with the development of stronger side plates for sliding screws and the combination of various medial displacement or valgus osteotomies with sliding rather than fixed devices.

One disadvantage of all three methods is the magnitude of the surgical procedure required for the successful completion of the method chosen. An extensive exposure of the proximal lateral femur is always required; the fracture site is frequently exposed and manipulated under direct vision; extensive muscle dissection is required in order to expose a sufficient area of the lateral femur to permit application of the surgical device; and some resection and manipulation of bone is essential if an osteotomy is performed. All of these surgical maneuvers have a significant effect in increasing the morbidity of the surgical procedure in the elderly patient.

In 1970 Kuntscher (24) advocated fixation of trochanteric fractures of the femur via an approach completely different from any of those previously mentioned. The concept was that of intramedullary fixation using a curved, rigid, 10-mm nail introduced at the medial femoral condyle over a guidewire. It was hoped that such an approach would obviate the morbidity associated with a direct surgical approach on the fracture and still provide sufficient stability of the fracture site to permit early weight-bearing. A similar approach using multiple narrow diameter pins was described by Ender in 1970 (9).

The biomechanical principle of this technique is to reduce the bending moment exerted on the external fixation device by shifting the position of the device closer to the compression vector acting on the femur (11). The pins are thus less subject to bending stress and have better weight-bearing stability than any device applied to the lateral side of the femur. This was similar to the concept report by Kuntscher for his single 10-mm nail. The use of multiple flexible pins offered significant advantage over a single nail. No guidewire was required, the presence of multiple pins permitted fixation in the often osteoporotic proximal femoral segment, and by using a number of nails a snug fit of the nails within the medullary canal of the femur was ensured in even the most osteoporotic patients (18).

A number of articles appeared in the English literature shortly after Ender's in 1970 that promoted this concept and suggested that improved morbidity and mortality in elderly patients with intertrochanteric fracture of the femur could be achieved by this technique (1,2,4,6,10,13,18–21,23,26,30–32,34,39).

We began using this operative technique at St. Michael's Hospital in Toronto in 1976, and it soon became our conventional method of treatment of inter- and subtrochanteric fractures of the femur. We currently have experience in more than 600 patients with this method of treatment and find it eminently satisfactory in the great majority.

Rationale

The problems faced by patients with intertrochanteric fractures are depressingly repetitive. The patients are generally elderly, their bones are fragile because of osteoporosis, they cannot tolerate prolonged bed rest, and they lack sufficient coordination and mental agility to cooperate with complex nonweight-bearing regimens after surgery. The depressingly high mortality figures for patients with fractures of the proximal femur are related to all of the foregoing features (15).

It is believed therefore that the solution to this problem is an operation carried out within 24 hr of admission to the hospital under a short-lasting anesthetic to minimize anesthesia-related complications to the sensorium. A surgical approach is utilized which minimizes tissue trauma, muscle dissection, and blood loss, and a fixation device is implanted which permits early uncontrolled weight-bearing without fear of implant failure or penetration in osteoporotic bone. It is our experience in 600 patients which encourages us to believe that the operation of Ender is such a procedure.

Considerable detail in this chapter is devoted to the surgical technique and postoperative care. This is necessary because, as always when embarking on a new surgical technique, technical errors are frequent. It is unfair to the operation and the surgeon who designed it to attribute such technical errors to the technique itself rather than to the surgeon who performed the technically inadequate surgery. Further information on the surgical technique favored by the author is available in a teaching film from the American Academy of Orthopaedic Surgery.

Technique

Two essentials for this operation are an extension-type fracture table and an image intensifier. Under suitable anesthesia the patient is positioned on the fracture table, and the image intensifier is brought in from the lateral aspect of the patient. The unaffected limb is positioned in wide abduction to permit the surgeon to stand between the legs. The fracture is reduced by traction and slight internal rotation. An attempt should be made to overreduce the fracture into slight valgus. It is essential that a satisfactory reduction be obtained prior to Ender nailing. Failure to obtain reduction makes successful nailing extremely difficult.

Once fracture reduction has been obtained, nails of appropriate length should be chosen. The nails are 4 mm in diameter and come in a wide variety of lengths from 30 to 48 mm. To select a nail of appropriate length, an unsterilized nail should be placed along the anterior aspect of the patient's thigh with the distal end of the nail at the level of the adductor tubercle. With the image intensifier, the proximal end of the nail should be seen to lie at the cortex of the femoral head. Because some magnification of the nail length occurs by having the nail lying on the anterior aspect of the thigh, it is important that the nail appear slightly too long at the time of selection. Once the appropriate length has been determined, a minimum of four nails of appropriate length and four nails 1–2 mm shorter and 1–2 mm longer should be selected and autoclaved.

The distal thigh and proximal leg is then prepared with suitable antiseptic solution and the limb draped in such a way as to provide surgical access to the distal one-half of the thigh.

The femur is approached via a curvilinear incision parallel to the posterior border of the vastus medialis muscle. After the fascia overlying this muscle is incised, the entire muscle belly can be reflected anteriorly without dividing any muscle fibers. With the medial femur thus exposed, the superior metaphyseal branch of the medial geniculate artery is visible running from the posterior aspect of the femur in a subperiosteal position. This vessel marks the spot at which the femur should be broached. It is proximal to the medial femoral condyle. After cauterization of the vessel and reflection of the periosteum from the medial femur, a 0.25-inch drill hole is made through the cortex at this level. This hole should be located at the posterior aspect of the medial femoral cortex immediately anterior to the posterior cortex of the femur. The posterior location of the hole is important because it avoids interference with the patellar mechanism; it is placed close to the strong posterior bone of the distal femur, providing protection against the stress riser effect of the entry hole.

Once the drill hole is made, it should be progressively enlarged in a proximal direction with the use of an awl and rongeurs until an opening 1.5 cm in width and 2.5 cm in length is obtained. It should be generally oval in shape.

Once the entry hole has been satisfactorily formed, the first nail may be inserted. It is important to prebend the first one or two pins into moderate anteversion. Because the proximal femur is anteverted, it is important to antevert the first nails to prevent retroversion of the proximal fragment of the fracture as a consequence of posterior pressure on the proximal fragment by a straight nail (*12,29*). This anteversion is readily accomplished with the use of a small plate bender.

With the nail held firmly in the insertion device, it is pushed up from the opening in the distal femur as far as possible using manual pressure only. The nail generally travels to the isthmus of the femur before binding between the nail and the bone is sufficient to prevent further progress. With the use of the mallet, the nail is then driven up through the isthmus and across the fracture site into the femoral head. The progress of the nail across the fracture site and into the proximal femur should be observed on anteroposterior (AP) and lateral image intensification. The nail should be seated firmly within the femoral head past the equator of the head and within 4–5 mm of the subchondral bone. The distal end of the nail should still protrude distal to the entry hole

Intertrochanteric Femur Fractures 81

in the distal femur but should lie flush against the cortical bone. Subsequent nails are inserted in a similar fashion, and an attempt is made to fan the nails in the proximal fragment of the femur in both the AP and lateral planes in order to ensure maximum rotational stability of the fracture. Nails should not be permitted to fall through the entry hole into the medullary cavity of the femur because these nails do not provide support for the fracture.

An attempt should be made to completely fill the medullary cavity with pins in order to provide secure fixation of the fracture and prevent undue motion of nails within the medullary canal. A minimum of four nails are used in most elderly patients, and frequently five or six nails may be required. This "stacking" of the medullary canal is essential to prevent the nails from backing out and thus loss of fracture fixation.

Once all of the nails have been inserted, the wound is closed and a Jones bandage applied. We found that the Jones bandage is extremely helpful in preventing sympathetic knee effusion after this operation, and it does not prevent the patient from taking weight during the immediate postoperative period.

On the day after surgery the patient is encouraged to stand at the bedside, taking as much weight as possible on the affected leg. Progressive ambulation with assistance is encouraged from the first day. No attempt is made to maintain the patient's leg in traction or in any external splinting other than the Jones bandage. Once the patient is confident with his walking on a walker or parallel bars, he is progressed to crutches and then canes. The Jones bandage and sutures are removed in 10 days. The use of external aids is encouraged indefinitely and is mandatory until the fracture has healed. Healing is generally evident on x-ray by 8 weeks after the fracture in the form of abundant callus formation.

Complications

The complications of this procedure are generally related to lack of experience with the operation, and they diminish as experience with the technique is gained. General complications of any hip fracture (e.g., deep vein thrombosis, urinary tract problems, bronchopneumonia, and decubitus ulcers) in our experience are generally less common in these patients than with other methods of fracture management. We attribute this to earlier ambulation with this technique. Specific complications related to the technique of Ender nailing which we have encountered include the following: external rotation deformity, pin prominence at the knee, pin penetration through the femoral head, and supracondylar fractures of the femur (3,17,27,29).

External Rotation Deformity

External rotation deformity generally occurs as a consequence of failure to produce sufficient anteversion at the fracture site at the time of nailing. This may be prevented by prebending the nails into anteversion, thus preserving the anteversion angle restored by the initial reduction of the fracture. Only the first one or two nails should be anteverted because as more nails are passed straight nails may be placed in different quadrants of the femoral head more readily than prebent nails. Early weight-bearing also tends to promote correct orientation of the leg, and we have noted persistent external rotation problems only in those patients who are not ambulatory after fixation of their fracture.

Pin Prominence at the Knee

Pin prominence distally occurs for one of three reasons. If nails of improper length are selected, the distal end is unduly prominent. This can be prevented only by selecting the proper nail length. Pin prominence may also occur if the entry hole is placed too far anteriorly on the distal femur. Proper orientation of the hole is essential to prevent this complication. If undue prominence of the pins is noted at the conclusion of the nail procedure, these prominent ends should be bent in such a way as to direct them posteriorly and toward the medial femoral cortex, thus preventing interference with the overlying patellar mechanism. The third cause of pin prominence relates to excessive settling of the fracture site and distal extrusion of the nails. This is generally apparent within a few weeks of fracture fixation. This can be prevented by ensuring that the femoral canal is filled by the nails selected and that the nails are firm within the medullary cavity. Such stacking not only prevents pin prominence but prevents loss of fracture position caused by excessive settling of the fracture during ambulation.

Penetration of the Hip Joint

In our experience penetration of the hip joint has occurred only if the nails had been inadvertently introduced into the hip joint at the time of initial nail insertion. Should this occur, it is not enough to merely back the nail out of the hip joint; the nail must be entirely removed from the femur and reinserted in a different direction and into a different portion of the femoral head. Failure to replace the nail allows the nail to intrude into the hip joint with settling of the fracture. We are not aware of any patient in our series in which pin penetration of the joint occurred providing the head had not been broached at the time of nail insertion.

Supracondylar Fracture of the Femur

Supracondylar fracture may occur because of a stress riser effect of the hole in the medial femoral cortex. This tendency can be greatly diminished by ensuring that: (a) the hole is oval without sharp corners; (b) the hole itself is filled with the nails inserted; and (c) the hole is of adequate size initially so that crack propagation from the hole during nail insertion does not occur. Suitable care is necessary at the time of nail insertion to avoid excessive stress at the distal end of the femur in patients with osteoporosis (22).

The use of multiple flexible nails for the management of intertrochanteric fractures of the femur does not represent a panacea. In our experience, however, there is a substantial reduction in 6-month mortality for such patients compared to the conventional lateral approach and use of a sliding hip screw (15). There is also a significant reduction in morbidity, especially evident in patients with unstable intertrochanteric fractures. We have seen a reduction in the 6-month mortality—from 24% to 11%—and a subsequent reduction in morbidity especially compared to patients managed with medial displacement osteotomies for unstable intertrochanteric fractures (16).

There is an unfortunate tendency for this operation to be reserved for patients who would do badly with any surgical procedure: the elderly, disoriented, incontinent, nonambulatory patient with a difficult unstable intertrochanteric fracture of the femur. It is not surprising that if the operation is limited to patients of this type it will achieve a reputation of being a poor

Intertrochanteric Femur Fractures

operation with poor results. If the surgical procedure is utilized in all patients with intertrochanteric fractures of the femur by a surgeon with a good understanding of the technique involved and a willingness to modify his approach to the postoperative management of such patients, a gratifying improvement in postfracture morbidity and mortality can be achieved.

It remains our firm conviction that Ender nailing is a relatively simple operative procedure which has few and readily avoidable technical pitfalls. We believe that it offers a significant advantage over conventional nail plate appliances for intertrochanteric fractures and offers all of the advantages of the sliding screw plate or nail plate devices without the disadvantages associated with a direct surgical approach to the femur.

REFERENCES

1. Arpin H, Kilfoyle RM (1980). Treatment of trochanteric fractures with Ender rods. J Trauma 1:32–42.
2. Bohler J (1975). The Hip. Mosby, St. Louis, pp. 170–179.
3. Chan KM, Chan KT, Lee SY, et al. (1982). Complications in treatment of trochanteric fractures using Ender's nails—a review of 120 patients. Ann Acad Med Singapore 11:162–169.
4. Chapman MW, Bowman WC, Csongradi JJ, et al. (1981). The use of Ender's pins in extracapsular fractures of the hip. J Bone Joint Surg 63A:14–28.
5. Collado F, Vila J, Bertran BE (1973). Condylocephalic nail fixation for trochanteric fracture of the femur. J Bone Joint Surg 55B:774–779.
6. Corzatt RD, Bosch AV (1978). Internal fixation by the Ender method. JAMA 240:1366.
7. Dimon JH III, Hughston JC (1967). Unstable intertrochanteric fractures of the hip. J Bone Joint Surg 49A:440–450.
8. Ecker ML, Joyce JJ III, Kohl EJ (1975). The treatment of trochanteric hip fractures using a compression screw. J Bone Joint Surg 57A:23.
9. Ender J (1970). Probleme bei frischen per—Und subtrochanteren obeschenkel bruchen. Hefte Unfallheilkd. 106:2–11.
10. Hall G, Ainscow DA (1981). Comparison of nail plate fixation and Ender's nailing for intertrochanteric fractures. J Bone Joint Surg 63B:24–28.
11. Harris LJ (1980). Closed retrograde intramedullary nailing of pertrochanteric fractures of the femur with a new nail. J Bone Joint Surg 62A:1185.
12. Herrlin K, Esund N, Andersson S, Wall A (1982). Anteversion measurements in trochanteric fractures of the femur. Acta Radiol [Diagn] (Stockh) 23:409–413.
13. High J, Lund B, Lucht J (1981). Trochanteric and subtrochanteric fractures: the operative results in a prospective and comparative study of Ender nailing and McLaughlin osteosynthesis. Acta Orthop Scand 52:639–643.
14. Holt EP (1963). Hip fractures in the trochanteric region: treatment with a strong and early weight bearing. J Bone Joint Surg 45A:687–705.
15. Hunter GA (1974–1975). The results of operative treatment of trochanteric fractures of the femur. Injury 6:202–205.
16. Hunter GA, Krajbich I (1978). Results of medial displacement osteotomy. Presented at the Canadian Orthopaedic Association Meeting.
17. Iwesbu CG, Patel RJ (1981). Difficulties and complications of the Ender method of treatment of trochanteric fractures of the femur. Injury 13:116–124.
18. Jenson JS, Sonne-Holm S (1980). Critical analysis of Ender nailing in the treatment of trochanteric fractures. Acta Orthop Scand 51:817–825.
19. Jenson JS, Sonne-Holm S (1980). Unstable trochanteric fractures: a comparative analysis of four methods of internal fixation. Acta Orthop Scand 51:949–962.
20. Jenson JS, Tndevold E, Sonne-Holm S (1980). Stable trochanteric fractures: a comparative analysis of four methods of internal fixation. Acta Orthop Scand 51:811–816.
21. Jones CW, Morris J, Hirchowitz D, et al. (1977). A comparison of the treatment

of trochanteric fractures of the femur by internal fixation with a nail plate and the Ender technique. Injury 9:35–42.

22. Kolmert L, Persson DM (1980). Supracondylar femoral fractures as a complication to Ender nailing of trochanteric fractures: a new device for osteosynthesis. Arch Orthop Trauma Surg 97:51–55.

23. Kuderna H, Bohler N, Collon D (1976). Treatment of intertrochanteric and subtrochanteric fractures of the hip by the Ender method. J Bone Joint Surg 59A:604–611.

24. Kuntscher G (1970). A new method of treatment of pertrochanteric fractures. Proc R Soc Med 63:1120.

25. Kyle RF, Gustilo RV, Premer RF (1970). Analysis of six hundred and twenty-two intertrochanteric hip fractures. J Bone Joint Surg 61A:216.

26. Lee PC, Bons Sc, Chow SP (1982). The treatment of unstable trochanteric fracture by Ender's nailing—early results of a prospective trial. Ann Acad Med Singapore 11:162–169.

27. Levy RN, Sieseld M, Sedlin Ed, Siffert RS (1983). Complications of Ender pin fixation in basicervical, intertrochanteric, and subtrochanteric fractures of the hip. J Bone Joint Surg 65A:66–69.

28. Massie W (1962). Extracapsular fractures of the hip treated by impaction using a sliding nail plate fixation. Clin Orthop 22:180–202.

29. Olerud S, Stark A, Gillistrom P (1980). Malrotation following Ender nailing. Clin Orthop 147:139–142.

30. Pankovich AM, Trabishy IE (1980). Ender nailing of intertrochanteric and subtrochanteric fractures of the femur. J Bone Joint Surg 62A:635–645.

31. Passoff TL, Schein AJ (1980). Ender's flexible intramedullary pins for the treatment of pertrochanteric hip fractures: preliminary report of the first one hundred cases. J Trauma 10:876–879.

32. Rausstad TS, M Ister A, Haukeland W, et al. (1979). Treatment of pertrochanteric and subtrochanteric fractures of the femur by the Ender method. Clin Orthop 138:231–237.

33. Roberts A, Rooney T, Loupe J, et al. (1972). A comparison of the functional results of anatomic and medial displacement valgus nailing of intertrochanteric fractures of the femur. J Trauma 12:341.

34. Russin LA, Sonni A (1980). Treatment of intertrochanteric and subtrochanteric fractures with Ender's intramedullary rods. Clin Orthop 148:203–212.

35. Sarmiento A (1963). Intertrochanteric fractures of the femur 150-degree nail plate fixation and early rehabilitation. J Bone Joint Surg 45A:706–722.

36. Sarmiento A (1975). The Hip. Mosby, St. Louis, pp. 159–169.

37. Schatzker J, Waddell JP (1980). Subtrochanteric fractures of the femur. Orthop Clin North Am 11:539.

38. Schumpelick W, Jantzen PM (1955). A new principle in the operative treatment of trochanteric fractures of the femur. J Bone Joint Surg 37A:693–698.

39. Waddell JP (1980). Sliding screw fixation of proximal femoral fractures. Orthop Clin North Am 11:607.

Ipsilateral Hip and Femur Fractures: Methods of Treatment

7

Frank F. Cook
James C. Binski
Marshall Horowitz

Concomitant fractures of the hip and femoral shaft are relatively rare injuries, almost exclusively observed in the polytraumatized patient. Treatment of this injury complex has been variable. In previous series nonoperative treatment consisted of a period of traction followed by immobilization in a spica cast or cast brace. When operative treatment was employed, the hip and/or the femur fractures were stabilized with intramedullary nails, plates, sliding hip compression screws, Zickel nails, Knowles pins, or Ender nails, alone or in combination (1–5, 7,8,10,13,18,20,24,25). In some femoral neck fractures, muscle pedicle bone grafts were employed to facilitate healing. Of 88 ipsilateral hip and femoral shaft fractures reported in the English literature, good to excellent results were obtained in 54 (61%) patients.

Historical Review

The initial series of ipsilateral hip and femoral shaft fractures was reported by Delaney and Street in 1953 (4). Their series consisted of four basilar neck fractures and concomitant femoral shaft fractures. All their patients were involved in high-energy head-on vehicular accidents and sustained polytrauma, including ipsilateral knee injuries. In their initial two cases, the shaft fractures were stabilized with intramedullary nails; the neck fractures were overlooked. Subsequently, the neck fractures were identified on postoperative radiographs and treated with Knowles pins. The next two concomitant neck fractures were identified at initial presentation. These fractures were stabilized with Knowles pins in addition to intramedullary stabilization of the shaft fractures. All their patients achieved good results.

Kimbrough reported an additional five cases (10), in each of which the patient was a victim of a high-velocity head-on vehicular accident and sustained

85

polytrauma. Three of the patients with initial delay in diagnosis had less than optimal final results. The final two cases—a femoral neck-shaft fracture treated with the combination of a Smith-Petersen nail and traction and a pertrochanteric-shaft fracture treated in traction—achieved good results.

Dencker's series underscored the tremendous energy involved in producing simultaneous hip and femoral shaft fractures (5). Of eight patients, three died as a result of polytrauma sustained at the time of injury.

A pattern seems to have been established. The obvious femoral shaft fracture in the polytraumatized patient draws the surgeon's attention away from other underlying injuries. Often complete hip and knee examinations are not performed. Every major series reports at least one delay in diagnosis of the concomitant hip fracture. Combining all series, 22% of the hip fractures were overlooked on initial evaluation. Associated ipsilateral knee injuries are also common and occurred in 28% of the patients.

In Schatzker and Barrington's series of six patients, the two treated with internal fixation of both fractures achieved good results (20). Bernstein (2) reported that the majority of his patients with good results were treated by internal fixation of both fractures. Internal fixation of femoral shaft fractures was especially recommended in the presence of associated patellar fractures.

Casey and Chapman (3) reviewed 21 cases of this fracture combination. Ten patients achieved good results with internal fixation of both fractures. These authors stated that knee injuries were frequently responsible for residual disability, and in order to minimize this complication fixation of both fractures to

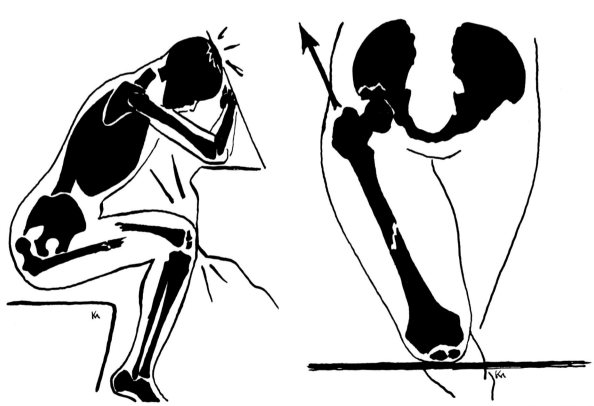

Figure 7–1 Pathomechanics of the dashboard femoral fracture.

Figure 7–2 With the hip in adduction, the femoral head is not well covered by the acetabulum. The resulting injury is hip dislocation with a shaft fracture.

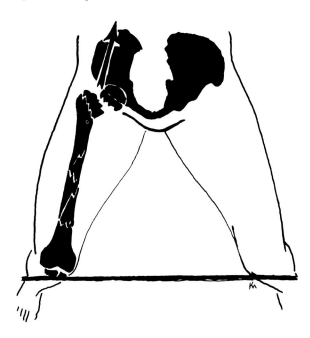

Figure 7–3 With the hip in abduction, the femoral head is firmly seated in the acetabulum. The resulting injury is fracture of the hip and shaft.

permit early range-of-motion exercises was recommended. This method of treatment prevents intraarticular changes from prolonged immobilization (6).

Zettas and Zettas (25) reported an additional 12 patients, seven of whom achieved full hip and knee motion with fixation of both fractures.

Pathomechanics

Concomitant hip and femoral shaft fractures occur as the result of very high kinetic energy transmitted to the bone (11,12). Every patient with this fracture combination was involved either in vehicular accidents or falls from considerable heights. The usual mechanism of injury involves a longitudinal compression force to the femoral shaft, the "dashboard" injury (18) (Figure 7–1). Initially, the transmission of forces through the knee region may result in significant local injury. Patellar fracture and/or ligamentous knee damage are common. If all the energy has not been dissipated in the subsequent femoral shaft fracture, fracture or dislocation of the hip results. The position of the femoral shaft at impact determines the type of hip injury. If the shaft is in adduction, dislocation will occur (Figure 7–2). If the shaft is abducted with the femoral head firmly seated in the acetabulum, fracture of the hip will result (Figure 7–3).

Management

After adequate treatment of life-threatening injuries, the polytraumatized patient must be thoroughly scrutinized for musculoskeletal injuries. The presence of a femoral shaft fracture should be an indication for careful examination of the hip and knee joints. The hip joint should be completely examined by radiographs. The presence of a knee effusion warns that ligamentous or intraarticular damage should be suspected (21,22). Instability of knee ligaments should be evaluated prior to the application of tibial pin traction. We concur with Walling

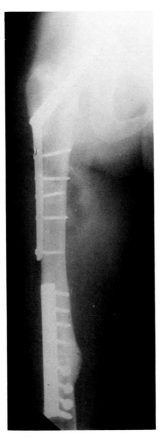

Figure 7–4 A pertrochanteric fracture and concomitant shaft fracture stabilized by a compression hip screw and compression plate with an autogenous bone graft. Both fractures united with unrestricted joint motion. The existence of a stress riser between the plates is recognized with this combination of fixation devices.

Figure 7–5 Bilateral basilar neck fractures and bilateral femoral shaft fractures. A Initial treatment of shaft fractures with compression plates. B Poor osteosynthesis on the left resulted in early fatigue and fracture of the plate.

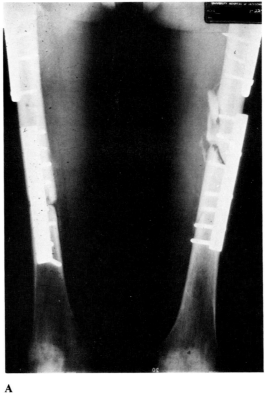

A

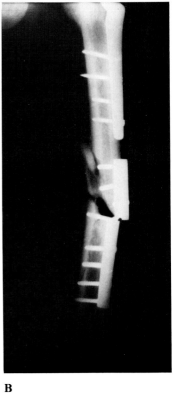

B

Ipsilateral Hip and Femur Fractures

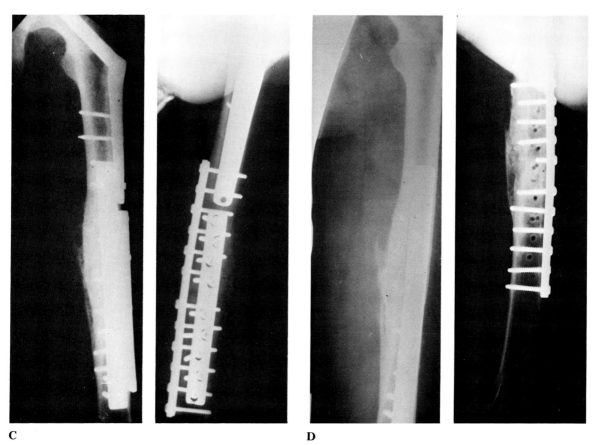

Figure 7–5 (cont.) C Loss of stabilization managed by application of dual plates and a bone graft. Note the anterior plate spanning gap between the lateral plate and Jewett nail side plate. **D** Both fractures healed; the Jewett nail and anterior plate are removed. Unrestricted joint motion was achieved.

et al. (22) in recommending the diagnostic use of femoral pin traction in this situation for evaluating knee ligamentous injury.

Open fractures should be immediately debrided and copiously irrigated. Depending on the status of the wound at this time, a decision can be made to proceed with immediate fixation of the fractures, or the injured extremity can be placed in traction. Definitive treatment by internal fixation can be performed at a later time depending on the condition of the wound and the absence of infection. Prophylactic antibiotics are always recommended.

The simplest method of stabilizing ipsilateral hip and femoral shaft fractures is the utilization of a sliding hip compression screw for the hip fracture and a separate compression plate for the shaft fracture (Figure 7–4). A potential complication is the presence of a stress riser between the two plates. Additionally, meticulous adherence to the principles of osteosynthesis must be observed. A plate stabilizing a femoral shaft fracture failed in one of our patients with bilateral hip fractures and bilateral femoral shaft fractures because medial cortex to cortex contact was not achieved, adequate proximal screw fixation of the plate was lacking, and a supplemental bone graft was not utilized (Figures 7–5A,B). The broken plate was removed and the fracture stabilized with anterior and lateral compression plates with a supplemental autogenous bone graft (Figure 7–5C). At last follow-up, the fracture had united with full hip motion and two of the surgical implants had been successfully removed (Figure 7–5D).

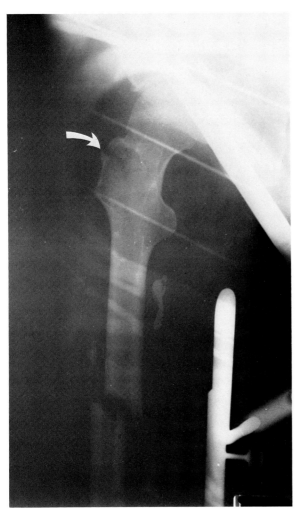 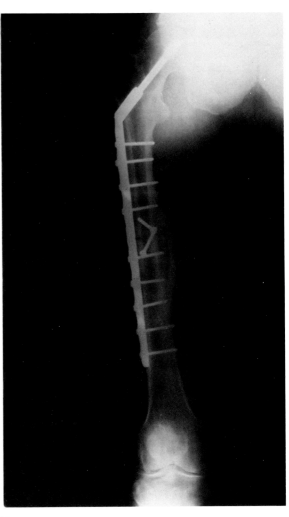

Figure 7-6A A 67-year-old male sustained a stable pertrochanteric fracture and a displaced transverse shaft fracture. Treatment consisted of internal fixation of both fractures using a single device. An autogenous bone graft was placed about the shaft fracture. **B** The result at 1 year shows both fractures united with unrestricted hip and knee motion.

If the shaft fracture is in the proximal half of the femur, both fractures may be spanned by a single device: a sliding hip compression screw with a long side plate (available by special request from Richards Medical Co. or Synthes) (Figures 7-6A,B). With combination femoral shaft and femoral neck fractures, the surgeon may stabilize the shaft fracture with an intramedullary nail followed by Knowles pin fixation of the neck fracture (Figures 7-7A,B).

Authors' Experience

We reviewed our experience in 11 patients with 12 ipsilateral hip and femoral shaft fractures. The majority of our patients suffered polytrauma from vehicular accidents. Four patients sustained ipsilateral knee injuries. All of the hip fractures were diagnosed on initial evaluation.

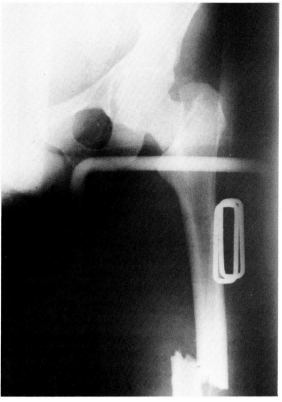 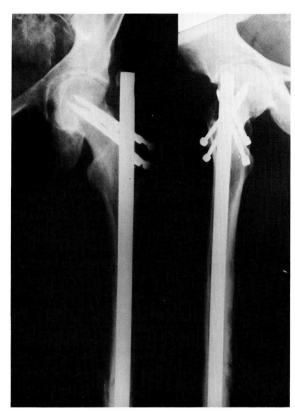

A   **B**

Figure 7–7A This 21-year-old male sustained a nondisplaced femoral neck fracture and a displaced transverse femoral shaft fracture in a motorcycle accident. **B** Both fractures primarily stabilized with an intramedullary nail and multiple Knowles pins. Both fractures healed, and the patient was fully ambulatory at 6 months.

There were five intracapsular and seven pertrochanteric hip fractures. The femoral shaft fractures were located in the mid-diaphysis in seven fractures, in the distal diaphysis in four, and in the supracondylar region in one. One supracondylar, one subtrochanteric, and two diaphyseal femur fractures were open. One patient sustained bilateral hip and bilateral femoral shaft fractures. Only one other patient with bilateral hip and shaft fractures had been previously reported (20).

Treatment of these injuries consisted of internal fixation of both fractures with the exception of one open femoral shaft fracture treated in traction and subsequent cast brace. No postoperative pulmonary complications or surgical infections were encountered.

With one exception, all fractures united with good to excellent results. One nonunion occurred in a femoral neck fracture which had been treated with poor stabilization (Figure 7–8). The associated ipsilateral femoral shaft fracture treated with an intramedullary nail united without incident. The patient currently functions well with a total hip replacement arthroplasty.

Results

All the reported cases of ipsilateral hip and femoral shaft fractures were reviewed and grouped according to treatment and final functional result (Table 7–1).

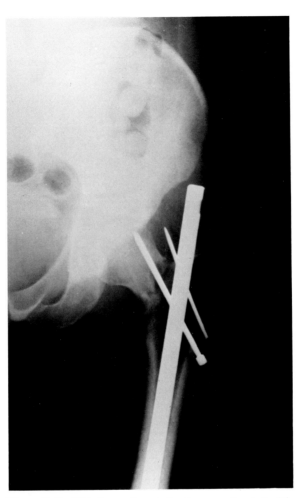

Figure 7–8 This femoral neck fracture was treated with a single Knowles pin and a Steinman pin to block rotation. Early loss of fixation occurred; the patient developed nonunion and aseptic necrosis of the femoral head.

Group A—internal fixation of both fractures
Group B—internal fixation of one fracture combined with traction and subsequent cast immobilization
Group C—Both fractures treated with traction and spica cast

The largest number of good results, 47 (89%), were in group A. The poor results in this group consisted of one death due to adult respiratory distress syndrome (ARDS), one infection, two hips with femoral head aseptic necrosis, and two patients with restricted hip mobility.

In Group B, there were only nine (41%) good results. Poor results in this group were mainly due to restricted motion in the hip or knee joints. Also, lack of recognition of the hip fracture on initial evaluation led to mal- or nonunion of that fracture.

In Group C, 16 patients were treated without internal fixation. All of the fractures in these patients were treated in traction initially. Some of the patients in the group were subsequently immobilized in a spica cast. Nine of

Ipsilateral Hip and Femur Fractures

Table 7–1. Ipsilateral Hip and Femoral Shaft Fractures

Series	Group A Internal fixation (good/poor)	Group B Internal fixation & traction (good/poor)	Group C Traction only (good/poor)
Delaney & Street (4)	4/0		
Ritchey et al. (18)		0/1	
Kimbrough (10)		1/2	1/1
Dencker (5)	3/2	0/1	0/2
Schatzker & Barrington (20)	2/0	1/2	0/1
Mackenzie (13)		1/3	
Horowitz (8)	1/0	0/1	
Bernstein (2)	6/1	1/2	1/2
Wolfgang (24)	1/0		
Ashby & Anderson (1)	3/0		
Casey & Chapman (3)	10/1	2/0	7/1
Zettas & Zettas (25)	7/1	2/1	
Present series	10/1	1/0	
Total			
Good/poor	47/6	9/13	9/7
% Good	47/53 = 89%	9/22 = 41%	9/16 = 56%

16 patients (56%) achieved good results. Seven of the nine good results were reported by Casey and Chapman (*3*); however, these authors noted that all of the respiratory complications that occurred in their patients were confined to those treated in traction. None were seen in patients treated with internal fixation of both fractures and with immediate postoperative mobilization. As a result of their experience, they recommended internal fixation of both fractures in this injury (*3*).

Classification and Preferred Treatment

Obviously, the individual surgeon's experience should dictate the type of internal fixation that is used in treating ipsilateral hip and femoral shaft fractures. Figure 7–9 depicts a method of classification for this injury complex based on the type of hip fracture: intracapsular, stable pertrochanteric, and unstable pertrochanteric fractures. It is further subdivided by the extent of the femoral shaft fracture: stable or unstable. Using this classification, a preferred method of treatment for these injuries is presented (Figure 7–9).

Type I-A: Femoral Neck Fracture and Stable Shaft Fracture

Author's choice: Knowles pins and intramedullary nail.

Initially, the shaft fracture is stabilized with an intramedullary nail by closed technique if possible (*23*). While the patient is still under biplane fluoroscopic control, Knowles pins are introduced anterior and posterior to the intramedullary nail and driven up the femoral neck into the head (Figure 7–7B). The presence of a basilar neck fracture is a contraindication to intramedullary fixation of the femoral shaft because proximal reaming may extend the fracture.

Success with flexible Ender nails introduced medially and laterally for fixation of the shaft fracture has been reported (*3,15*). However, Knowles pins must still be used for additional stabilization of the neck fracture. This technique may be useful in the presence of a basilar neck fracture. The presence of a distal shaft fracture is a contraindication for retrograde insertion of Ender nails.

I. FEMORAL NECK FRACTURE AND

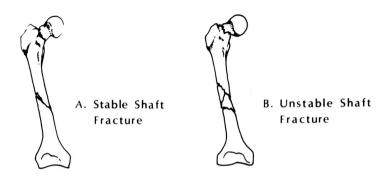

A. Stable Shaft Fracture   B. Unstable Shaft Fracture

II. STABLE PERTROCHANTERIC FRACTURE AND

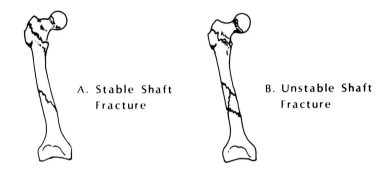

A. Stable Shaft Fracture   B. Unstable Shaft Fracture

III. UNSTABLE PERTROCHANTERIC FRACTURE AND

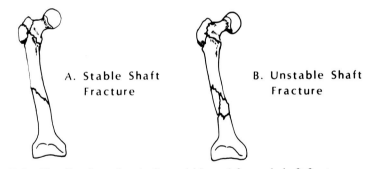

A. Stable Shaft Fracture   B. Unstable Shaft Fracture

Figure 7–9 Classification of an ipsilateral hip and femoral shaft fracture.

An alternative method of treating this injury combination is to stabilize the shaft fracture with a compression plate supplemented with an autogenous bone graft and fix the femoral neck fracture with a sliding hip compression screw.

Type I-B: Femoral Neck Fracture and Unstable Shaft Fracture

Authors' choice: Knowles pins and compression plate with autogenous bone graft.

In the presence of a comminuted shaft fracture, compression plating and bone grafting is the most reliable method of treatment in our hands. However, intramedullary fixation with supplemental cerclage wires and a bone graft may

Ipsilateral Hip and Femur Fractures

be used. Surgeons experienced with the Grosse-Kempf interlocking intramedullary nail may wish to utilize this technique for stabilization of severely comminuted shaft fractures with a loss of bone stock. A period of postoperative traction may be required in the more comminuted fracture.

Type II-A: Stable Pertrochanteric Fracture and Stable Femoral Shaft Fracture

Author's choice: Sliding hip compression screw with long side plate.

The stable pertrochanteric fracture and proximal shaft fracture is best treated with a sliding hip compression screw with a long side plate (Figure 7–6B). The pertrochanteric fracture is initially stabilized with a compression hip screw. This presents no problem in the undisplaced fracture. In the displaced fracture, however, an open reduction is required after the proximal shaft has been exposed. The side plate of the compression hip screw is left unattached to the proximal shaft fragment until the shaft fracture has been reduced. The reduction is maintained with bone clamps or temporary cerclage wires while the plate is secured to the proximal shaft with cortical screws. The large AO compression device is then used to compress the shaft fracture, after which the side plate is secured to the distal shaft fragment. In all cases an additional autogenous iliac bone graft is placed about the shaft fracture.

Ender nails may be employed in treating stable pertrochanteric fracture patterns. As described by Olerud and others, anteversion of the Ender nails should be employed to prevent malrotational deformities (14,16). The technically proficient surgeon may choose to stabilize the pertrochanteric fracture with a sliding hip compression screw and use Ender nails for stabilization of the shaft fracture. We have no experience with the difficult procedure of passing Ender nails beyond the plate screws of the hip compression device (15,17).

Type II-B: Stable Pertrochanteric Fracture and Unstable Femoral Shaft Fracture

Authors' choice: Sliding hip compression screw with long side plate and bone graft.

The presence of an unstable shaft fracture complicates the achievement of stable internal fixation. Additional forms of stabilization are always required, e.g., interfragmentary fixation with lag screws and the use of cerclage wires. In all instances, bone grafting must be performed with care taken to place most of the graft along the medial side of the fracture. A period of postoperative traction may be required. We cannot recommend the use of Ender nails in the unstable femoral shaft fracture.

Type III-A: Unstable Pertrochanteric Fracture and Stable Femoral Shaft Fracture

Authors' choice: Proximal stabilizing procedure, sliding hip compression screw with long side plate, and autogenous iliac bone graft.

The unstable pertrochanteric fracture should first be rendered stable by either a valgus osteotomy described by Sarmiento (19) or a medial displacement osteotomy popularized by Dimon and Hughston (9). Then internal fixation of the shaft fracture with a long side plate is accomplished as outlined previously. Again, intramedullary nailing of any type is not recommended in the treatment of this fracture combination.

Type III-B: Unstable Pertrochanteric Fracture and Unstable Femoral Shaft Fracture

Authors' choice: Proximal stabilizing procedure, sliding hip compression screw with a long side plate, supplementary internal fixation, and bone graft.

This fracture combination represents the most complex injury to treat by internal fixation. All of the methods of internal fixation mentioned in the previous types may be necessary. Ideal stability still may not be achieved, and a period of skeletal traction followed by nonweight-bearing, either in a wheelchair or on crutches, may be required.

Summary

The following points should be reemphasized:

Our experience, coupled with a review of the literature, confirms that internal fixation of both hip and ipsilateral femoral shaft fractures allows early hip and knee motion. In addition, immediate postoperative mobilization of the patient is possible, decreasing pulmonary complications.

Surgeons evaluating femoral shaft fractures must thoroughly examine the hip and knee joints for occult fractures and/or ligamentous injuries which may otherwise go unrecognized.

In our opinion, internal fixation of both fractures is the treatment of choice.

A method of classifying these complex injuries is presented and the preferred treatment modalities discussed.

Acknowledgments

The authors would like to thank Ms. Shirley Branch and Ms. M. E. Wofford for their secretarial assistance. We also thank Gladys DonAroma, Stephen Englert, Mark Hildreath, and Daniel Kent for their patience and technical expertise. We are indebted to Drs. Robert Kleinhans and Hugh Switzer for their radiographs and suggestions.

REFERENCES

1. Ashby ME, Anderson JC (1977). Treatment of fractures of the hip and ipsilateral femur with the Zickel device: a report of three cases. Clin Orthop 127:156–160.
2. Bernstein SM (1974). Fractures of the femoral shaft and associated ipsilateral fractures of the hip. Orthop Clin North Am 5:799–818.
3. Casey CJ, Chapman MM (1979). Ipsilateral concomitant fractures of the hip and femoral shaft. J Bone Joint Surg 61A:503–509.
4. Delaney MM, Street DM (1953). Fracture of femoral shaft with fracture of neck of same femur: treatment with medullary nail for shaft and Knowles pin for neck. J Int Coll Surg 19:303–312.
5. Dencker H (1965). Femoral shaft fracture and fracture of the neck of the same femur. Acta Chir Scand 129:597–605.
6. Enneking MF, Horowitz M (1972). The intra-articular effects of immobilization on the human knee. J Bone Joint Surg 54A:973–985.
7. Fielding JM, Cochran GVB, Zickel RE (1974). Biomechanical characteristics and surgical management of subtrochanteric fractures. Orthop Clin North Am 5:629–650.
8. Horowitz T (1972). Ipsilateral fractures of the femoral shaft and neck associated

with patellar fracture and complicated by entrapment of a major intermediate fragment within the quadriceps muscle: a report of two cases. Clin Orthop 83:190.

9. Hughston JC (1974). Intertrochanteric fractures of the femur (hip). Orthop Clin North Am 5:585.

10. Kimbrough EE (1961). Concomitant unilateral hip and femoral shaft fractures—a too frequently unrecognized syndrome: report of five cases. J Bone Joint Surg 43A:443–449.

11. Kulowski J (1956). Etiology of motorist injuries. Clin Orthop 7:246–252.

12. Kulowski J (1957). Concluding opinions: some orthopaedic aspects of motor-vehicle accidents. Clin Orthop 9:331–344.

13. Mackenzie DB (1971). Simultaneous ipsilateral fracture of the femoral neck and shaft: report of eight cases. S Afr Med J 45:459–467.

14. Olerud S, Stark A, Gillstrom P (1980). Malrotation following Ender nailing. Clin Orthop 147:139–142.

15. Pankovich A, Goldflies M, Pearson R (1979). Closed Ender nailing of femoral shaft fractures. J Bone Joint Surg 61A:222–232.

16. Pankovich A, Tarabishy I (1980). Ender nailing of intertrochanteric and subtrochanteric fractures of the femur. J Bone Joint Surg 62A:635–645.

17. Pankovich A, Tarabishy I, Barmada R (1981). Fractures below noncemented femoral implants. J Bone Joint Surg 63A:1024–1025.

18. Ritchey SJ, Schonholtz GJ, Thompson MS (1958). The dashboard femoral fracture: pathomechanics, treatment and prevention. J Bone Joint Surg 40A:1347–1358.

19. Sarmiento A (1975). Valgus osteotomy technique for unstable intertrochanteric fractures. In: The Hip Society. Mosby, St. Louis.

20. Schatzker J, Barrington TW (1968). Fractures of the femoral neck associated with fractures of the same femoral shaft. Can J Surg 11:297–305.

21. Walker DM, Kennedy JC (1980). Occult knee ligament injuries associated with femoral shaft fractures. Am J Sports Med 8:172–174.

22. Walling AK, Seradge H, Spiegel PG (1982). Injuries to the knee ligaments with fractures of the femur. J Bone Joint Surg 64A:1324–1327.

23. Weller S, Kuner E, Schweikert CH (1979). Medullary nailing according to Swiss study group principles. Clin Orthop 138:45–55.

24. Wolfgang GL (1976). Combined trochanteric and ipsilateral shaft fractures of the femur treated with the Zickel device: a case report. Clin Orthop 117:241–246.

25. Zettas JP, Zettas P (1981). Ipsilateral fractures of the femoral neck and shaft. Clin Orthop 160:63–73.

Preoperative Planning of Corrective Surgery for Posttraumatic Deformities in the Adult

8

Jeffrey W. Mast
William A. Teipner
Aaron A. Hofmann

Recently there has been increased interest in the methods used by Pauwels (4), Blount (1), Mueller (3), and others to preoperatively plan the outcome of operations for acute fractures or reconstructive procedures on the bones and joints of the extremities. This interest has been nurtured by the evolution of better means of obtaining reliable internal fixation of fractures and osteotomies. Internal fixation is enhanced when it is planned in advance. The optimum location of lag screws and the proper dimensions of plates or nails may be accurately depicted, avoiding loss of time in surgery because of this type of decision-making. Additional benefits are derived from the mental process that goes into the plan as the steps of the operation are developed and the problems to be encountered are evident in advance of the actual procedure. The final result obtained in the plan may be compared to the sound joint or limb, and relatively exact data regarding the effect of the surgery can be seen, e.g., changes in length, effects on the mechanical axis of joints, and the presence of any significant displacement of the anatomic axis of the operated limb.

When planning we must consider six possible corrections (2). There are three possible angular deformities: (a) in the frontal plane, varus and valgus; (b) in the sagittal plane, flexion and extension; and (c) in the horizontal plane, external rotation and internal rotation. There are also three displacements: (a) in the frontal plane, medial and lateral; (b) in the sagittal plane, anterior and posterior; and (c) shortening or lengthening. Preoperative planning lends itself easily to evaluation of malalignment in the frontal and sagittal planes. Thus angular deformities and displacements are easily rendered, but rotational malalignment must usually be determined clinically and corrected at the time of surgery.

We may describe deformities as simple, existing in only one plane; compound, existing in two planes; or complex, existing in all three planes. Any of these deformities may be associated with one or more displacements. Correction

99

of a deformity is ideally concerned with all aspects of it and should include both angulations and displacements.

The object of this chapter is to present the technique of preoperative drawings the authors use in carrying out indicated corrections of deformities residual to trauma. It is a method that has been refined through many discussions with Professor M. E. Mueller of Bern, Switzerland. Examples of deformities of the distal femur are used for illustrations of the points found in the text.

Materials

Two radiographs—an anterior-posterior (frontal plane) and lateral (sagittal plane)—taken with good technique and a standard distance of 40 inches must be available of both the malaligned extremity and the normal side. In the lower extremity it is occasionally necessary to obtain a full length axis view in order to appreciate the mechanical axis of the limb. If this is not available, the physiological mechanical axis may be used and corrections carried out using these angles as a guide (Figure 8–1). A viewbox with good illumination is used as a

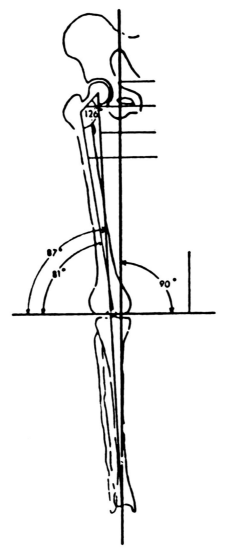

Figure 8–1 The limb axis. The mechanical axis is a line passing through the center of the hip, knee and ankle. In the distal aspect it corresponds to the anatomic axis of the tibia. It converges with the vertical axis at an angle of 3° distally. The normal anatomic axis of the femoral shaft converges with the mechanical axis at the knee joint at an angle of 6°. The knee joint axis is perpendicular to the vertical axis and stands at an angle of 81° with femoral shaft axis and 87° with the tibial shaft axis.

Posttraumatic Deformities

drawing board. This is preferably placed horizontally on a table top to facilitate tracing the contours of the x-ray. One viewbox, Mediview (Protek, Indianapolis, Indiana) is extremely well suited to this purpose. In addition, an abundance of tracing paper is necessary. We recommend Monroe triple T parchment tracing paper, 14 × 17 inches, as it is transparent enough and large enough to use in most circumstances.

Multiple colored felt tip pens and a goniometer round out the necessary items. The goniometer is extremely important, and the authors' personal preference is a model designed by Professor Mueller and distributed by Protek. The aim of the correction is to produce a limb that is as close as possible to the uninjured or normal side. The planning is therefore based on the sound side.

Methods

A tracing is made of the x-ray of the normal side in the anteroposterior (AP) or frontal plane and is compared to the physiological axis to see if there are preexisting abnormalities in the normal extremity. A tracing is also made of the corresponding view of the bone with the deformity. The tracing of the deformed bone is then superimposed on that of the normal bone by turning the tracing over and aligning the proximal portions. The axis of the proximal "normal portion" is then drawn onto the tracing of the deformed bone. Where the contours of the bones depart from one another is likewise marked. The same procedure is then carried out on the distal portion of the bone by overlapping the distal contours. The normal axis is marked in the deformed distal fragment, drawing it in as it was with the proximal fragment. The external contours of the bone are matched, and where they depart is marked on the drawing of the deformed bone. The same procedure is carried out for the other x-ray view. Thus the axes and the point at which the external contours of the bone deviate from one another are marked on the tracing of the deformed bone. The derivation of the correction usually starts in the plane in which there is the greatest deformity, but it sometimes commences in the other planes because of convenience or a fixed limitation. Using the marks where the contours of the bones leave one another as reference points, two fragments can be developed. In most cases the points match or approximately match on the drawings made from each set of x-rays (AP and lateral). Each fragment contains the anatomic axis as it was previously traced from the normal. Each fragment is then traced on an individual paper along with its axis. When this has been completed a reduction of the two fragments is carried out by appropriate manipulation of the papers. The anatomic axes are made to match, and the mechanical axis of the adjacent joint is made correct. Another piece of paper is placed over the two pieces that represent the reduction, and a tracing of this composite is made. The same procedure is carried out in the other plane. These are the tracings of the final correction. This tracing may be superimposed on the x-ray of the normal side, and residual discrepancies are visualized, including residual shortening. If the result of superimposition of the corrected side and the normal side is congruent, it is accepted. However, many times at this stage it may be seen that there is another problem (e.g., length) that is not satisfied, or that the contours of the bone deviate too much from the normal side. In this case the original two fragments must be remanipulated, or perhaps two different fragments are derived from the original tracings. After retracing two fragments separated at a different level, the same process is repeated in such a way that the optimum correction may be seen.

During the time of the manipulation of the two fragments on their separate pieces of paper, the type of osteotomy needed to accomplish the desired end result can be appreciated. Simple deformities are usually corrected by an opening or closing wedge which may be made perpendicular to the anatomical axis or at varying angles to it depending on the requirement for optimum length and fixation. Compound deformities are obviously more demanding, and their correction depends in which two planes the deformity exists. If the deformity is present in the frontal and sagittal planes, then both can usually be corrected by a transverse osteotomy if there is no length discrepancy. A steep oblique osteotomy may be used if some length is to be regained. If length is a major problem, a step cut osteotomy may be necessary. Complex deformities require correction in all three planes and are the most difficult to manage. A step cut osteotomy is the easiest means of solving the problem because it leaves osteotomy surfaces perpendicular to the anatomic axis, which affords the most reliable means to correct the torsional malalignment, although a trade-off between shifting the anatomic axis and providing good surface areas of contact is usually present.

Having arrived at the drawing of the final correction, the fixation is planned. This is done with the use of implant templates available through Protek. The desired implant is overlaid on the final correction and in its optimum location is traced into the composite. Critical screws for fixation are included. This completes the tracing of the final result. Dimensions such as the distance from

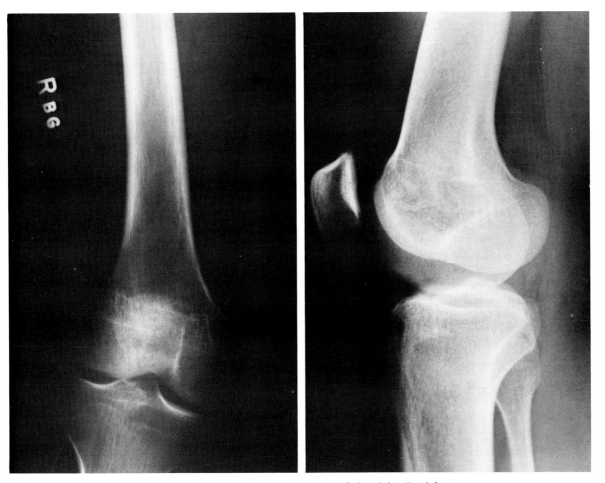

Figure 8–2A AP and lateral x-rays of the right distal femur.

Posttraumatic Deformities

the joint line to the end of the implant and the direction of screws and their measurements should be written in the margins of the drawing.

There remains only to develop the surgical tactic. This is rendered on the tracing of the original deformity using the intermediate steps that comprised the method of obtaining the final correction drawing. The steps of the operation are numbered; the location of the osteotomy is measured from a known landmark along with its inclination relative to a perpendicular to the anatomic axis of the bone or, alternatively, at a known distance from Kirschner wires placed parallel to a Kirschner wire placed along the axis of the adjacent joint. During surgery 2.0- mm Kirschner wires serve as guides for the correction, being inserted at the proper location according to the tactical drawing.

Examples

Simple Deformity

T.K. is a 30-year-old male with pain in the right knee. He had a history of fracture of the right distal femur at age 14. He was treated nonoperatively, and there was union of the fracture with valgus of the distal femur and clinical shortening of 1 inch (Figure 8–2).

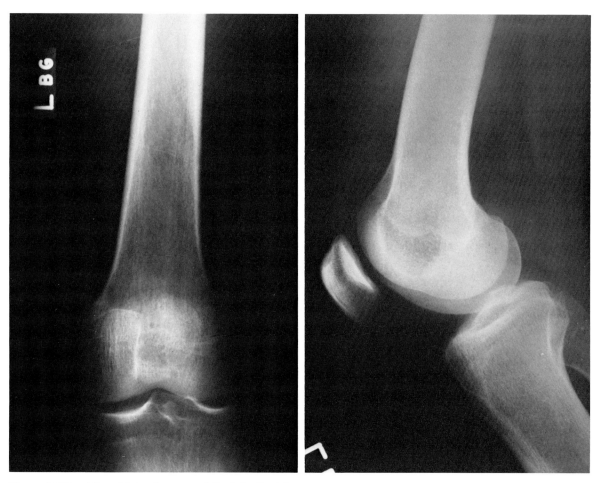

Figure 8–2B AP and lateral x-rays of the left distal femur.

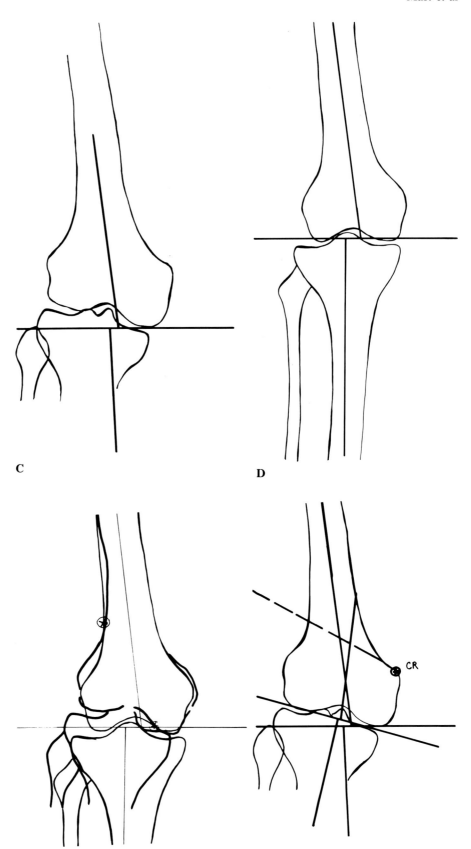

C

D

E

Posttraumatic Deformities

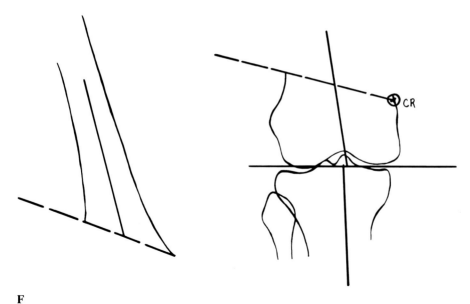

F

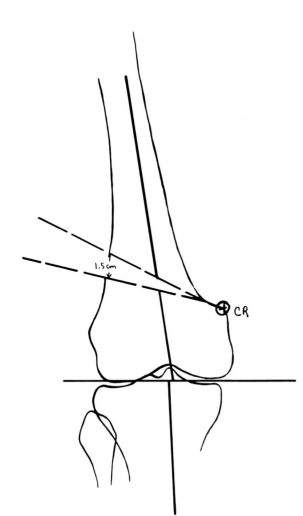

G

Figure 8–2C Tracing of the right distal femur in the frontal plane.

Figure 8–2D Tracing of the left distal femur in the frontal plane with superimposition of the physiological axis of the knee.

Figure 8–2E Superimposition of the left femur on the right. At this point the residual deformity is limited to the lateral 75% of the distal femur, and correction of this abnormality may restore the anatomic axis of the bone and result in restoration of mechanical axis of the knee. One can appreciate where the contours of the distal femur deviate on the lateral side, and this may be marked on the tracing. It is interesting that the contours on the medial side do not deviate. By superimposition matching the contours proximally the anatomic axis of the patient can be placed in the tracing of the proximal fragment. We can see that at a point 7 cm from the joint line on the lateral side an osteotomy can be based that would allow opening of only the lateral distal femur to restore the correct condylar relationships without disturbing the medial cortical margin. The largest surfaces for contact of an interpositional graft would be provided by an oblique osteotomy which would also be benefited by having the medial hinge in the transitional thin cortex of the diaphysis.

Figure 8–2F Two fragments can be created at these points complete with their correct anatomic axis.

Figure 8–2G The fragments are manipulated until the anatomic axes match and the mechanical joint axis is correct. This drawing is the final correction. By using a template of a 95° condylar blade plate, the proper sized implant and location of the screws may be added.

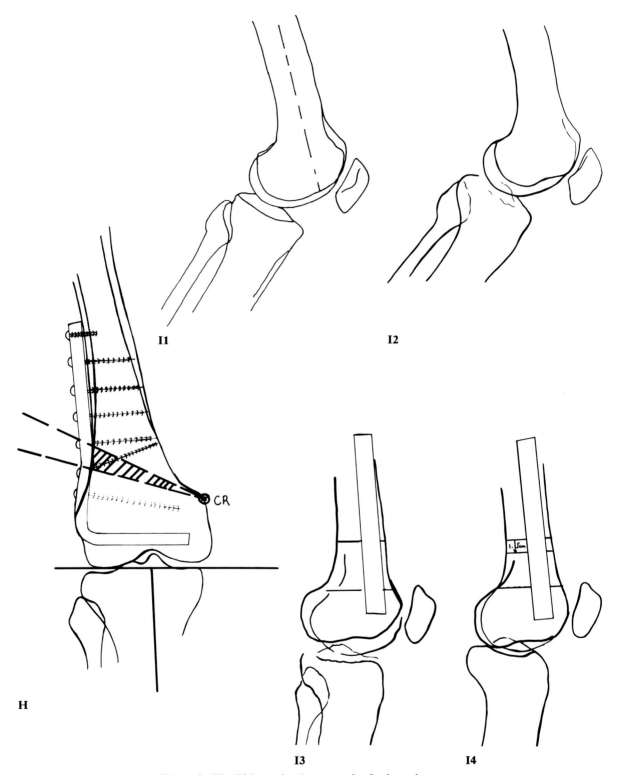

Figure 8–2H This tracing becomes the final result.

Figure 8–2I Since the length of the opening along the lateral cortex is known in the frontal plane, the drawings can be made in the sagittal plane, allowing lengthening of the silhouette of the lateral condyle of the femur the same distance from the osteotomy site distally, in this case 1.5 cm.

Posttraumatic Deformities

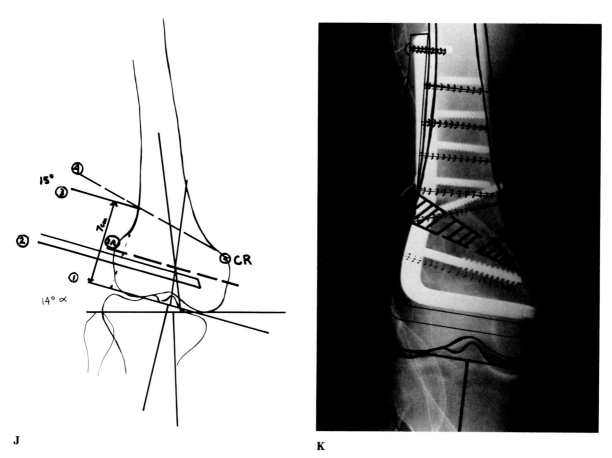

Figure 8–2J The surgical tactic is outlined on the drawing of the deformity. It is now possible to know the surgical exposure, the location of the osteotomy, the inclination of the osteotomy and how to find it, the size of the triangular bone graft to be taken from the iliac crest, the location of the seating chisel from the joint line. Additionally, because of the use of the fixed-angle blade plate, the articulating tensioner may be used to open the osteotomy once the cuts have been made. In this way instability should never become a problem (1) A 2.0-mm Kirschner wire through the joint which is in the orientation of the distal femur in the frontal plane. (*1a*) A 2.0-mm Kirschner wire on the anterior face of the joint condyles which is the orientation of the distal femur in the horizontal plane. (2) The insertion of the seating chisel which is located 1.5 cm from the joint line parallel to Kirschner wire (*1*) and parallel to Kirschner wire (*1a*). (3) A 2.0 mm Kirschner wire parallel to (*1*) plus (*2*) and 7 cm from the joint line. (4) The angle of obliquity of the osteotomy, in this case a 15° angle to (*3*). All of these reference points may be found at surgery with the use of an angled template guide and a ruler.

Figure 8–2K Final result with a superimposed drawing.

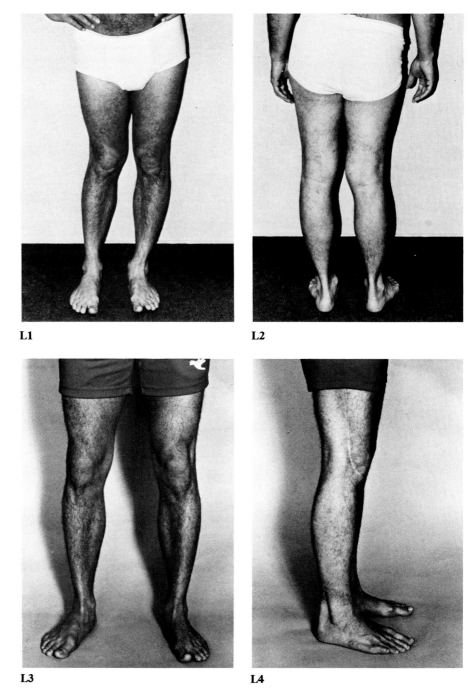

L1   **L2**

L3   **L4**

Figure 8–2L Clinical photographs before and 1.5 years after surgery. The patient has full restoration of function.

Compound Deformity

W.K. is a 42-year-old male who had a history of a severe conjoint supracondylar and intracondylar right femur fracture in 1974. The patient originally was treated with open reduction and internal fixation of his fracture. Fixation was lost, however, and the patient healed with valgus, external rotation, and posterior displacement. The patient had pain in the knee in the medial compartment and was clinically short 1 inch (Figure 8–3).

Posttraumatic Deformities

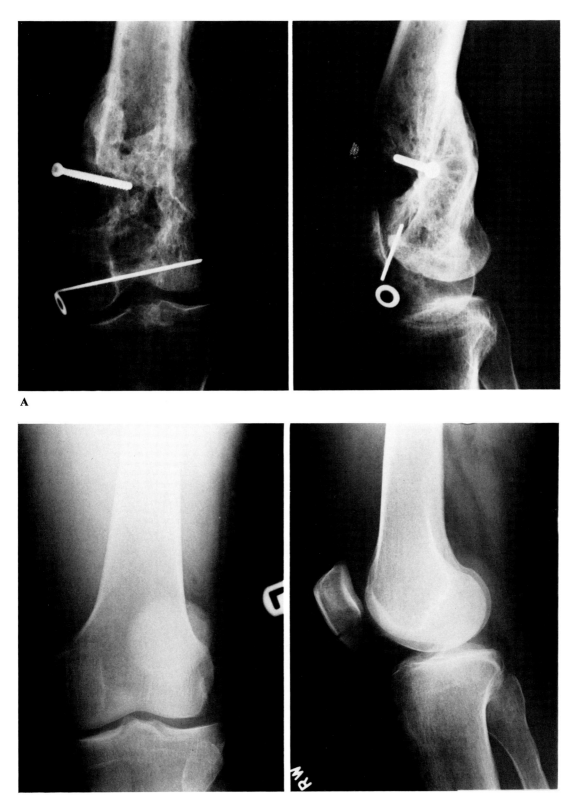

A
B
Figure 8–3A AP and lateral views of the right distal femur. **B** AP and lateral view of the left distal femur.

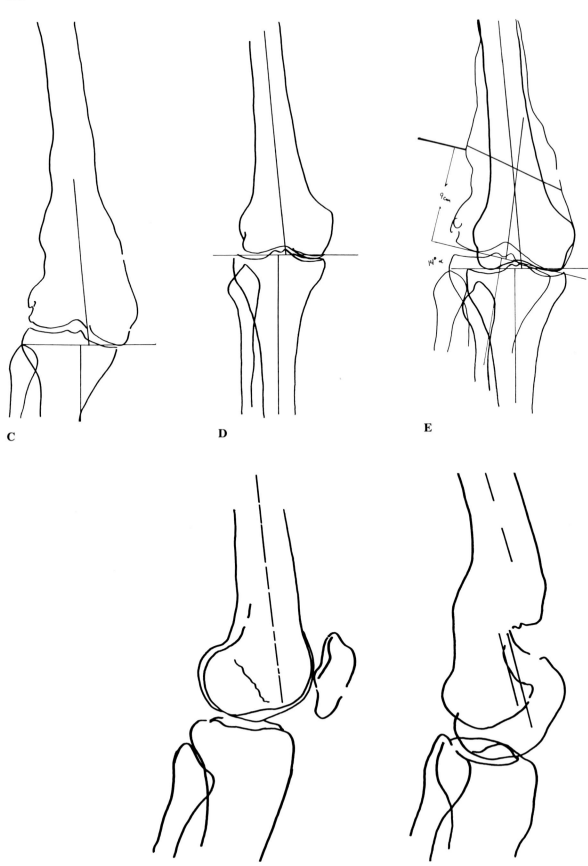

Posttraumatic Deformities

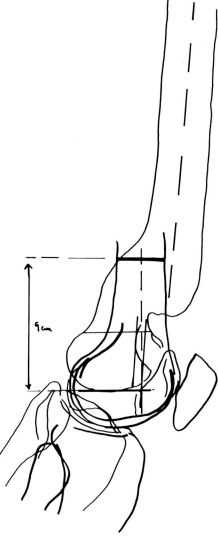

Figure 8–3C Tracing of the right femur in the frontal plane.

Figure 8–3D Tracing of the left femur in the frontal plane.

Figure 8–3E Superimposition of the right and left femurs in the frontal plane.

Figure 8–3F Tracing of the right and left distal femurs in the sagittal plane.

Figure 8–3G Superimposition of the right and left femurs in the sagittal plane. In this case the sagittal plane shows the variable which is the limiting factor for the level of the osteotomy. This is because of the posterior displacement of the lateral distal femur. Obviously if this is to be corrected, the osteotomy must be made within the confines of this fragment. The length of the old fragment appears to be 9 cm.

Figure 8–3H Two fragments then may be created, each containing, as in the first example, the anatomic axis of the femur based on the normal side. The length of the distal fragment along the lateral cortex is 9 cm. The inclination of the line of separation is somewhat arbitrary, and different slopes may be explored to see which appears to be the most satisfactory. In this case an inclination of 10° to the parallel of the end of the distal femur in the frontal plane is selected.

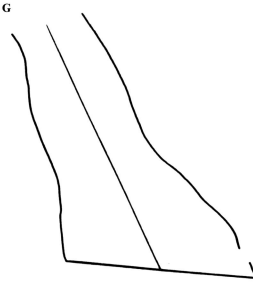

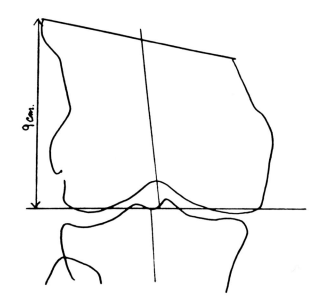

Figure 8–3I These two fragments are manipulated until the anatomic axis overlaps and the corresponding mechanical axis of the joint is correct. A composite drawing is then made. This is the drawing of the correction in the frontal plane.

Figure 8–3J As with the other example, since the lengthening of the lateral side of the distal femur is now known, a tracing of the correction in the sagittal plane may be made. By separating the two major distal fragments and redrawing the lateral condyle silhouette on a third piece of tracing paper, it may be lengthened independently of the medial side. This is true because the medial fragment in the frontal plane does not change in length. The anatomic axis in the sagittal plane is matched, and the lateral condylar tracing is moved distally the same amount as the lengthening obtained in the frontal plane. The discrepancy between the anatomic axis of the medial and lateral femoral condyle represents a rotational malalignment. This may be corrected on the drawing by aligning all axes, but at surgery it will be determined clinically and corrected by proper insertion of the seating chisel in the distal fragment.

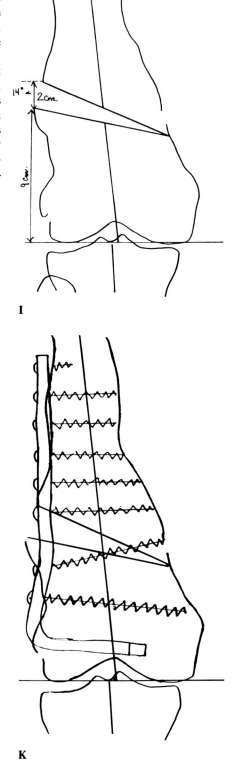

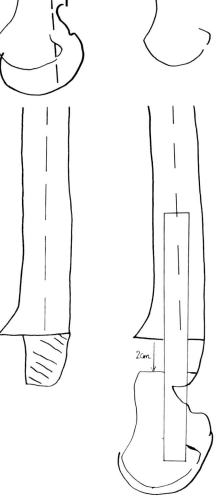

J   K

Posttraumatic Deformities

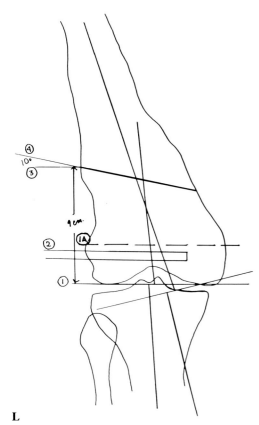

Figure 8–3K The appropriate implant may be selected from the template overlay and traced into the drawing of the final correction in both frontal and sagittal planes.

Figure 8–3L The surgical tactic is then drawn on the tracing of the original deformity. (*1*) A 2.0-mm Kirschner wire placed through the knee joint parallel to the axis of the distal femur in the frontal plane. (*1a*) The Kirschner wire placed along the anterior face of the distal femoral condyle representing the torsion of the distal fragment. (*2*) The insertion of the seating chisel 1.5 cm proximal to the joint line and parallel to Kirschner wires (*1*) and (*1a*) and to the anatomic axis of the distal fragment in the sagittal plane. (*3*) A Kirschner wire 9 cm from the joint line parallel to (*1*) and (*2*). (*4*) The desired inclination of the osteotomy relative to Krischner wire (*3*) in the frontal plane, in this case 10°.

Figure 8–3M Final x-rays with superimposition of the preoperative plan.

L

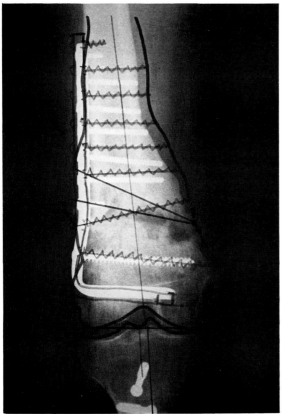

M1

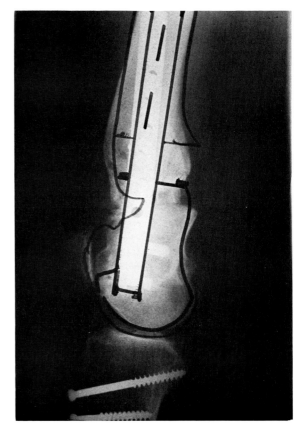

M2

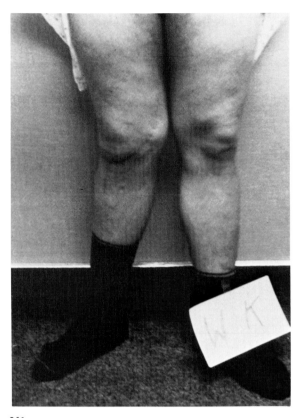

N1

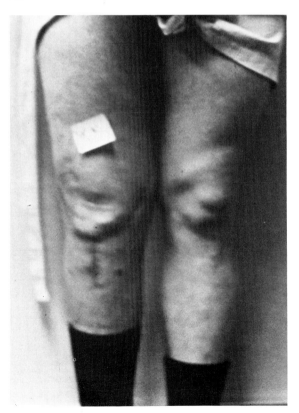

N2

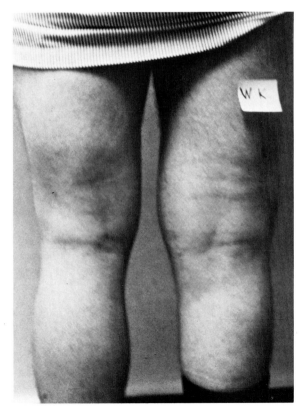

N3

Figure 8–3N Clinical photographs of the patient before and after surgery. The final range of motion on this patient is 100° of flexion and full extension.

Posttraumatic Deformities   115

Results

Eight patients with posttraumatic deformities of the distal femur have been
treated with supracondylar osteotomy of the type illustrated. A closing wedge
type osteotomy was utilized in five, whereas the correction was accomplished
in three via opening wedges depicted in the examples. In this small group of
cases all corrections were complete in that postoperative correction of the axes
allowed superimposition of the drawing of the final result on the final x-rays
in the appropriate plane with complete congruence of the cortical shadows.
Although final superimposition of the exact fixation devices is theoretically possible with careful adherence to the preoperative plan, it seems more difficult to
achieve as there are frequently small variations encountered at surgery that
influence placement of the implant and therefore lead to a sight postoperative
discrepancy between the drawing of the final result and the x-ray. This has
not been a problem because the discrepancies have been minor, usually consisting
of a difference in the length or inclination of a screw or a slight variation in
the level of location of the implant.

Discussion

The methods described are not only applicable in the distal femur but, using
the same sequence of planning, have been of value to us in corrections of posttraumatic deformities of all long bones. This is true for the upper as well as the
lower extremity. Recently, with the evolution of total joint surgery, there has
been more emphasis on the knowledge and maintenance of normal limb axes.
These considerations are also pertinent to the correction of posttraumatic deformities because the ideal situation is to be able to restore a deformity to normal
in all aspects. With a detailed plan one is able to see beforehand if it is feasible
to correct all aspects of the deformity and to delineate the surgical steps necessary
to carry out such a procedure successfully. One of the problems encountered
in discussing this form of planning is that the process itself is one of discovery.
As one proceeds through the various tracings one starts to understand exactly
what the problems are in the specific case and then can creatively play with
the possibilities on paper. If the solution becomes apparent during this process,
it must be asked if the solution is reasonable, i.e., that it does not violate some
basic biologic, surgical, or mechanical principle. It must also be worked out
as a surgical tactic, and if it is then possible to resolve the solution in a series
of simple steps the surgical execution becomes feasible. This results in a marked
improvement in the execution of the surgical procedure to the mutual benefit
of both patient and surgeon.

Summary

A general method of preoperative planning for correction of residual posttraumatic deformities has been discussed and presented by examples of planning
corrections of posttraumatic deformities of the distal femur; the method is applicable to posttraumatic deformities of the extremities in general, and it is emphasized that the method is of most value in the delineation of the problems so
that different solutions to the problem may be tested and criticized visually,
comparing them to the normal side. When this discovery process is complete,
if there are no basic biological, surgical, or mechanical rules violated a surgical

tactic may be developed by back-tracking through the steps used to obtain the tracing of the desired corrective result. These steps may then be followed at the time of surgery to carry out an operative procedure with a predictable outcome from the standpoint of correction of the deformity and stable fixation once the correction has been achieved.

REFERENCES

1. Blount WP (1964). Osteotomy in the treatment of osteo-arthritis of the hip. Bone Joint Surg 46:1297–1325.
2. Mueller ME (1973). Intertrochanteric osteotomy in the treatment of the arthritic hip joint. In: Surgery of the Hip Joint, edited by Tronzo RG. Lea & Febiger, Philadelphia, pp. 627–643.
3. Mueller ME (1979, 1980, 1983). Personal communications.
4. Pauwels F (1976). Biomechanics of the Normal and Diseased Hip. Springer-Verlag, New York.

Femur Fractures with Simultaneous Knee Ligament Injuries

9

Arthur K. Walling
Houshang Seradge
Phillip G. Spiegel

Because of the difficulty in diagnosis, the incidence of ligament injuries in the knee occurring simultaneously with ipsilateral femoral shaft fractures is unknown. Pedersen and Serra (2) first made this observation in a report of six cases in 1968, and an additional four cases were discussed by Shelton et al. (3) in 1971. With only 10 reported cases appearing in the literature prior to 1971, the frequency of these combined injuries seems to be small. However, a study by Dunbar and Coleman (1) in 1978 reported 14 of 20 patients (70%) who had at least minimal but definitely asymmetrical ligamentous laxity and five of 20 patients (25%) who had significant laxity. A similar experience was noted by Walker and Kennedy (4) from Canada in 1980, when they retrospectively reviewed 52 patients with femoral fractures, 48% of whom demonstrated knee ligament damage, 30% of these being of a severe nature. Twenty-three of the 26 injured knees in their study were not documented during their initial hospitalization. The latter two reports (1,4) challenge the assumption that knee ligament injuries occurring with ipsilateral femur fractures are infrequent. It is our intention to further document the incidence of these combined injuries and to present a practical method of diagnosing these injuries accurately and promptly.

Material

Twenty-four consecutive patients with femoral shaft fractures were prospectively examined during the 6-month period from 1 January 1978 to 30 June 1978 at Tampa General Hospital, University of South Florida Medical Center. No patient with a diaphyseal noncondylar fracture of the femur was excluded, and both open and closed fractures were included. The youngest patient was 14 years old and the oldest was 68; the average age was 23 years. The knee ligament

Table 9–1. Mechanisms of Injury

Type of accident	No. of patients	No. of patients with knee ligament injury
Motorcycle	10	6
Automobile	6	
Pedestrian vs. automobile	7	2
Bicycle vs. automobile	1	

Table 9–2. Ligament Involvement

Ligament involved	No. of patients
Anterior cruciate	3
Posterior cruciate	1
Lateral collateral	1
Anterior cruciate, posterior cruciate, lateral collateral and contralateral, lateral collateral	1
Anterior cruciate, medial collateral	2

injuries were diagnosed by history, physical examination, and roentgenographic studies that utilized specialized knee stress films and follow-up films of the knee if it was placed in traction.

Early in the study four patients were also evaluated with a single-contrast arthrogram. This was later discontinued because the diagnostic yield was low and the injury was better demonstrated by stress testing. Arthroscopy was not used because it was our intention to develop a diagnostic protocol that could be instituted in an emergency room without the need for a general anesthetic.

Of the 24 patients in the series, eight (33%) had sustained an injury to the ligaments of the ipsilateral knee. Eighteen patients were male, and six were female; of the eight patients with ligament injuries, six were male. The mechanisms of injury accounting for the femoral shaft fractures are listed in Table 9–1. It should be noted that the ligament injuries occurred in unprotected circumstances, where the patients sustained severe and, for the most part, multiple injuries.

The associated injuries in the eight patients with involvement of the knee consisted of a closed traumatic injury to the head in five, a visceral injury (ruptured spleen and contusion of the liver) in two, and a pelvic fracture in two. All eight patients had at least one additional major fracture.

Of the 16 patients without a ligament injury, eight had a closed traumatic injury to the head, one had a ruptured spleen, two had a pelvic fracture, and nine had at least one additional major fracture.

Once injury to the ligaments of the knee was diagnosed, an operation was done to stabilize the femur in four patients, and repair of the knee ligament was done in three of them. The five injured knees that were treated nonoperatively were protected during traction therapy for the fractured femur. A summary of the involved ligaments in the eight patients with femur fractures and associated knee injuries is given in Table 9–2.

Discussion

For prompt recognition of an injury to the knee ligaments in a patient with an ipsilateral femoral shaft fracture, one must strongly suspect the existence of the combined injury. During the physical examination, attention is naturally focused on the deformed, painful thigh; but in order to avoid overlooking a simultaneous ligament injury, the physician must include a careful local assessment of the ipsilateral knee. Specifically, any joint-line tenderness, areas of abrasion, lacerations, and ecchymosis are noted, and the presence or absence of

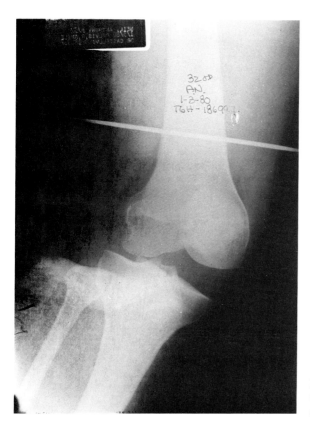

Figure 9-1 Method of distal femoral stabilization and stress testing.

effusion is recorded. As pointed out by Pedersen and Serra (2), ecchymosis and effusion may or may not be present initially but can occur several days after injury. If the knee swells after the initial evaluation or while the patient is in traction, it should be regarded as presumptive evidence of a significant knee injury and not be dismissed as effusion secondary to traction irritation or "sympathetic effusion." It is also important to examine the contralateral knee, as such involvement has been reported and was present in one of our patients.

The diagnosis of instability of the knee ligaments is made by stressing the involved ligament to determine the amount of laxity present and documenting the extent of the instability by obtaining x-rays of the joint while under stress (Figure 9-1). However, in the presence of a fracture of the femur with an unstable thigh, conventional methods of examining the knee are quite difficult to use. A Lachman's test may assess anterior-posterior stability, but in cases of subtle injury or when combined with varus-valgus instability it is impossible to stabilize the femur sufficiently to quantitate conventional examinations. In these instances, we recommend utilizing a distal femoral pin, as used in femoral traction, to achieve the femoral stability needed for stress testing. A medium-sized Steinman pin with a tension bow attached allows an assistant to control the distal femur. Having achieved femoral stabilization, the surgeon is free to manipulate the leg and obtain stress views of the knee ligaments in anterior-posterior and medial-lateral planes (Figure 9-2). If abnormal motion is detected, options for operative or nonoperative treatment of both injuries can be selected. We recommend the diagnostic use of a femoral stabilizing pin in all patients who have a fractured femur as a result of high-energy trauma as well as multiple injuries, especially closed traumatic injury to the head. In patients with injuries

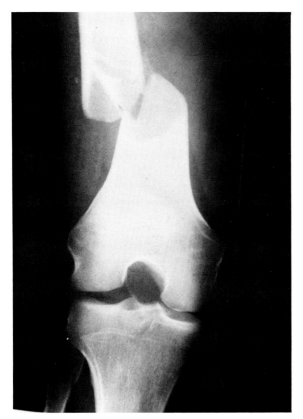 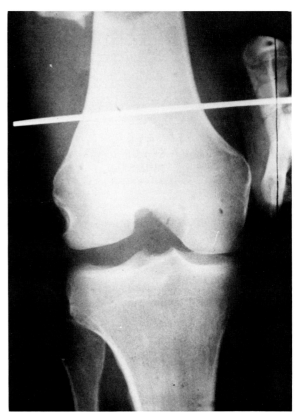

Figure 9–2A Anteroposterior view of a ligamentous injury in a 28-year-old male.

Figure 9–2B Varus stress view of the knee utilizing distal femoral pin stabilization defining the ligamentous injury.

caused by low-velocity trauma but with associated signs about the knee, e.g., ecchymosis, point tenderness, and effusion, the stabilizing pin should also be used.

Although it is our personal bias that combined femur and knee injuries present a relative indication for primary rigid fixation of the femur to allow treatment of the knee injury, we have developed a plan that allows several treatment options, depending on physician preference and patient circumstances at the time of diagnosis (Table 9–3). If our femoral stabilization pin is placed and ligament instability is demonstrated, and if primary fixation of the femur is elected, the femoral pin is removed and fixation carried out. It is believed that temporary sterile insertion of this pin does not compromise an open reduction and internal fixation, and the surgeon may then select treatment for the accompanying knee ligament injury. In the cases demonstrating ligament injury for which operative treatment of the femur is not elected, we have retained the femoral pin for traction and protected the knee ligaments from further damage by means of a plaster cast extending from the toes up to and including the femoral traction pin.

For obvious reasons, proximal tibial traction should never be used when it has been demonstrated that a femoral fracture and an injury to the knee ligaments coexist. If no abnormal knee motion is detected during stress testing and nonoperative treatment for the fracture is elected, the femoral stabilizing pin may be removed and a tibial pin can be utilized for traction.

Table 9-3. Treatment Plan Options

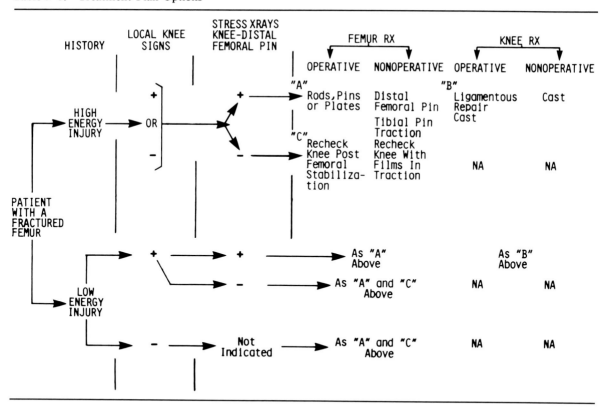

Follow-up x-rays of the knee in traction are recommended for all patients with femoral fractures treated by proximal tibial skeletal traction. Prior to our utilization of femoral pin stabilization for stress testing, routine traction views taken to include the knee demonstrated anterior subluxation or asymmetrical joint widening in four patients with femoral shaft fractures (Figure 9-4). On further evaluation, these patients were found to have unrecognized ligament injuries. We thus recommend that x-rays of patients in traction for femoral shaft fractures should include the knee in both planes, especially if there is any doubt concerning ligamentous integrity during the initial evaluation. Likewise, we reemphasize that the delayed appearance of an effusion during traction should prompt further evaluation for a ligamentous injury. Furthermore, should the femur have operative stabilization, the ipsilateral knee should be evaluated after stabilization in every case prior to the discontinuance of anesthesia (Figure 9-3).

Femoral stabilization using the pin traction method was especially advantageous in the multiply-injured patient with significant head trauma. Thirteen of the 24 patients we examined had sustained closed injury to the head, and five of them were shown to have an injury to the ligaments of the knee. These patients were unable to cooperate with the routine history-taking and physical examination and, because of their head injuries, were often not considered operative candidates. Femoral pin stabilization provided an easy method of diagnosing knee injury in these difficult-to-examine patients and provided a method of treatment that avoided further ligamentous damage by inappropriate traction methods.

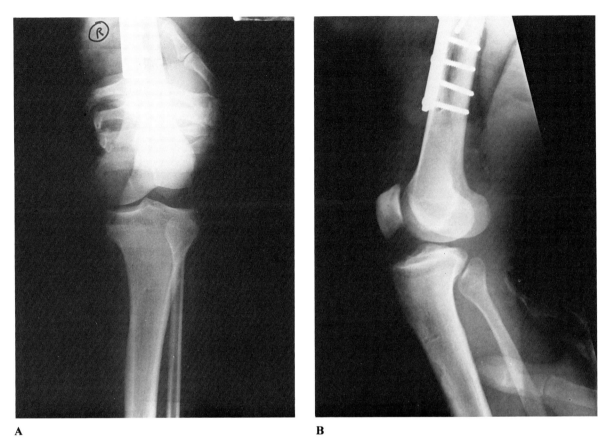

Figure 9–3 Grade II open segmental fracture of the right femur in a 31-year-old male. **A** This intraoperative varus stress radiograph of the knee was made after femoral stabilization. Intraoperative anteroposterior stress radiograph of the knee made after femoral stabilization.

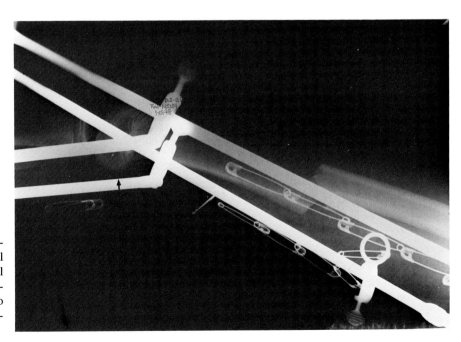

Figure 9–4 Fractured femur treated with proximal tibial traction. This lateral x-ray shows anterior displacement of the tibia to the femur indicating ligament injury (*arrow*).

Conclusions

This study focuses attention on the unrecognized incidence of ligament injuries to the knee that occur simultaneously with ipsilateral femoral shaft fractures, the need for early diagnosis, and a practical approach to follow in achieving that diagnosis. By maintaining a high index of suspicion, conducting a gentle but thorough physical examination, and utilizing diagnostic stress x-rays of the knee as well as follow-up views in traction, these concomitant injuries can be identified and a rational treatment plan instituted.

REFERENCES

1. Dunbar WH, Coleman SS (1978). Occult knee injuries associated with ipsilateral femoral fractures, a prospective study. Orthop Trans 2:253.
2. Pedersen HE, Serra JB (1968). Injury to the collateral ligaments of the knee associated with femoral shaft fracture. Clin Orthop 60:119–121.
3. Shelton MD, Neer CS, Grahtham SA (1971). Occult knee ligament ruptures associated with fractures. J Trauma 11:853–856.
4. Walker SM, Kennedy JC (1980). Occult knee ligament injuries associated with femoral shaft fractures. Am J Sports Med 8:172–174.

Dislocation of the Knee in the Competitive Athlete

10

J. R. Steadman
James B. Montgomery

Knee dislocation is a rare but severe injury associated with extensive soft tissue damage. It is a true surgical emergency. Vascular as well as neurologic injuries are commonly associated with the acute musculoskeletal trauma. Although the literature is replete with different opinions regarding the treatment of the ligamentous components (4,5,7,9), there is complete agreement on vascular lesions (1,2). The lack of dislocation when the patient is first seen at the hospital can also mean that a dislocation was identified and reduced at the scene of the accident. The highest incidence of knee dislocations occurs in motor vehicle accidents; knee dislocations also frequently occur in persons participating in soccer, football, skiing, and other sports.

Results of treatment for knee dislocations are divided into excellent, good, fair, and poor categories. Athletic participation mandates that the athlete attains an excellent or near-excellent result after the injury. Requirements of an athlete must be considered. For example, stiffness in the knee would eliminate those athletes who participate in sports involving the lower extremity, and intraarticular adhesions that provide some degree of static stability are unacceptable. Therefore a plan must be developed which addresses the static stability, flexibility, proprioception, dynamic protection, and endurance of the muscles across the knee joint. Static stability is important in maintaining the integrity of the joint over years of stress. Short-term return followed by degenerative changes in later years should be avoided. The combination of elasticity, proprioception of the joint, plus strength, power, and endurance of the muscles across the joint are all factors in regaining the physical ability to participate in competitive sports.

This chapter describes a proven method for obtaining optimal results for the athlete. The competitive athlete has a great personal commitment to return to sport(s) activity. An acceptable result in the general population may be unacceptable in the athletic population.

125

Classification

Dislocations about the knee are classified into five types: anterior, posterior, medial, lateral, and rotatory. The type of dislocation indicates the direction of the tibial shift in relation to the femur.

Kennedy (3) showed that hyperextension causes anterior dislocation in cadaver specimens. Posterior dislocations are caused by crush injuries or direct force on the tibia, forcing it posteriorly on the femur, e.g., a dashboard injury in an automobile accident. Direct or indirect violence produces other types of dislocations, i.e., lateral by valgus, medial by varus, and rotatory by rotatory forces.

Surgical Anatomy

The ligamentous anatomy of the knee should be understood thoroughly. The less obvious areas of injury during surgical treatment require attention because of their importance in postoperative stability of the knee after dislocations. These areas include the posterolateral corner, the popliteal muscle, and the patellar tendon. In addition, the orientation of the ligaments (e.g., the anterior cruciate, posterior cruciate, and posterior oblique ligament) must also be considered in the surgical treatment. One of the major advances in treatment of knee dislocation is appreciation of the value of the meniscus. Meniscus repair has enhanced success in the repair of knee dislocations.

A complete dislocation of the knee is accompanied by disruption of the soft tissue, all ligaments plus the popliteal tendon, the meniscus (menisci), and frequently the articular cartilage. Arterial and neurovascular damage may be associated with the dislocation.

The collateral circulation about the knee after dislocation is poor. The popliteal artery, which traverses the popliteal fossa, is anchored both proximally above the femur at the adductor hiatus and distally by a fibrous arch over the soleus muscle. The popliteal artery gives off five genicular arteries as it traverses the space. Although these have anastomoses with anterior tibial recurrent arteries, they may not provide adequate blood supply to maintain the viability of the leg (2). The tibial and common peroneal nerves which cross the popliteal area are not fixed as firmly as the artery. Therefore there is less chance of these nerves being injured than the vascular structures.

Diagnosis

The diagnosis of knee dislocation is made on both clinical and radiographic appearances (Figure 10–1). Clinically a deformity should be easily palpated. The hyperextension injury, with dislocation anterior to the tibia, is palpable under the skin. With the anterior dislocation of the knee, the femoral condyles are prominent posteriorly. With posterolateral dislocation, the medial femoral condyle is markedly prominent on palpation. Swelling may be absent upon palpation about the knee, and this should not rule out a dislocation. With tearing of the capsular structures, the blood from the knee joint may dissect into the soft tissues above and below the knee. With the popliteal artery injured, there may be marked swelling of the posterior popliteal area (Figure 10–2).

On radiographic analysis of the knee one may see bony avulsion of the ligamentous insertions about the knee, as well as gross instability on examination

Knee Dislocation

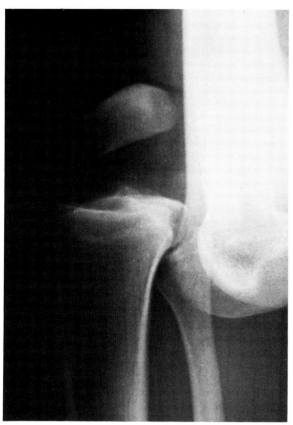

Figure 10–1 Lateral roentgenogram demonstrating anterior dislocation of the knee. The popliteal artery and vein were ruptured.

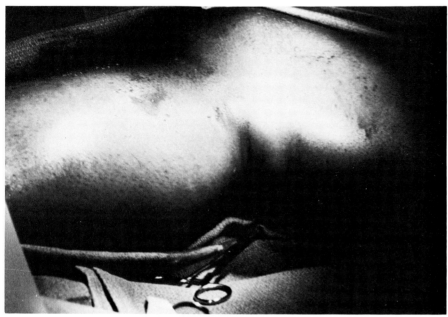

Figure 10–2 Reduced knee dislocation before surgery. The popliteal space is tense secondary to swelling with popliteal artery rupture after anterior dislocation.

of the knee. An unreduced dislocation is easily diagnosed by radiographic evaluation.

The posterior tibialis and dorsalis pedis pulses should be evaluated immediately. If they are not normal, the lower extremity should be positioned differently and the circulation reevaluated. If pulses are absent on palpable examination, a Doppler apparatus should be used. A warm but pulseless foot is not indicative of vascular sufficiency.

Neurologically, it is difficult to ascertain whether ischemia or injury to the peroneal or tibial nerve is causing dysfunction. Loss of cutaneous sensation, especially in the digits, suggests critical ischemia. It is extremely important, when examining a patient, not to cause any more damage. The extremity should be handled with caution.

Complications

Complications of traumatic dislocations of the knee are common and serious. Collateral circulation in a posttraumatic dislocation of the knee is poor and markedly impaired secondary to the severe trauma. With the two most frequent types of knee dislocations, anterior and posterior, there is about a 40% chance of an associated arterial injury (2). (Figure 10–3). Debakey and Simeone (1), in a review of arterial injuries during World War II, found an amputation rate of 49.6% when vascular flow was disrupted. With immediate reestablishment of blood flow (2), the amputation rate was decreased to 11.1% during the Korean War.

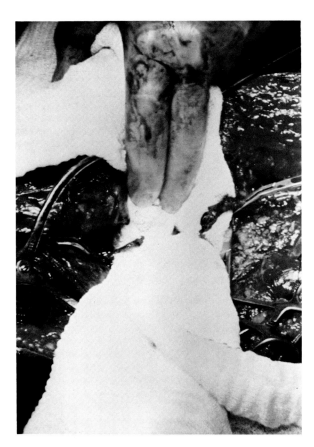

Figure 10–3 Popliteal artery at exploration with complete rupture and retraction of both ends.

Knee Dislocation

Lateral displacement of the tibia may impair the ability to reduce a knee dislocation. This may be secondary to inturning of the torn medial ligament or buttonholing the medial ligament above the medial femoral condyle. Neurologic injuries are most common in the peroneal nerve secondary to stretch and are most frequently associated with medial dislocations.

Treatment

Immediate treatment should consist of closed reduction as quickly as possible. The knee should not be hyperextended because hyperextension puts more tension on the already stretched vascular structures and nerves. Prompt reduction helps restore circulation and lessens the chance of nerve injury secondary to stretching. Anterior dislocations are reduced by longitudinal traction followed by pressure on the posterior femur, lifting it into the reduced position. One should not push the tibia posteriorly because hyperextension may aggravate the injury to the popliteal vessels. Posterior dislocation is reduced by longitudinal traction, extension of the knee, and lifting the proximal tibia. Lateral and medial dislocations are reduced by longitudinal traction and appropriate pressure on the tibia and femoral area.

After reduction, the neurovascular status of the knee should be thoroughly evaluated. The knee then should be immobilized in approximately 15°–30° of flexion with a splint or cast brace. A cast brace offers the advantage of being in place for use during the immediate postoperative period.

Circulation should be constantly monitored after the reduction. If an arterial pulse is not palpable, a Doppler apparatus should be utilized. A warm pulseless foot is not an indication of viability of the muscles and subcutaneous tissues. If the pulses are not present, arteriography or surgical exploration and repair should be undertaken (Figures 10–3 through 10–5). If an arteriogram is performed, it should be an expeditious (i.e., emergency) procedure. If the location of the lesion is known, an arteriogram may give little additional informa-

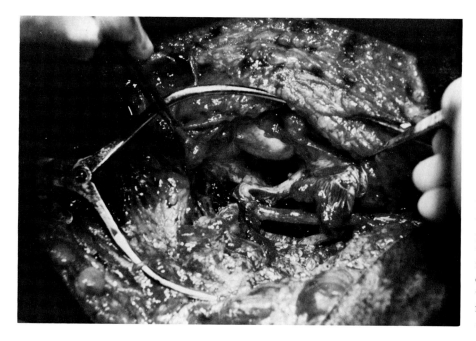

Figure 10–4 Wound after arterial and venous repair with a saphenous vein graft. Note the tearing of the posterior medial capsular structures with an exposed medial femoral condyle (*top center*).

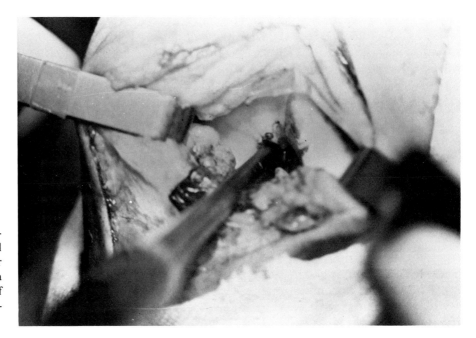

Figure 10–5 Surgical exposure of the femoral notch. The intercondylar notch was opened with a curette to allow repair of the anterior cruciate ligament.

tion, and so precious time would be lost by doing the procedure. Prolonging the treatment of the arterial injury beyond 6 hr after injury has a morbid effect on the end result (2).

Ligamentous injuries about the knee may be treated surgically or nonoperatively. Some surgeons (9) suggest that the knee should not be treated operatively because of the severity of the injury. Chances of obtaining good results from nonoperative treatment are possible. The likelihood of obtaining an excellent to near-excellent result, however, is unlikely.

Nonoperative treatment has been proposed by Mitchell (5), Myles (6), and others (9). Taylor et al. (9) reduced dislocations in a slightly flexed position; after reduction, quadriceps setting exercises were begun as soon as possible. Immobilization time averaged approximately 5.5 weeks. They stated that 18 patients treated nonoperatively had good results, and eight had fair or poor results. [Sixteen patients (among the total 42 cases) had some type of surgical procedure but could not be considered a "group" for comparison with the nonoperatively treated patients.] Although this may be an acceptable degree of success in the general population, it would not be considered acceptable in the athletic population.

O'Donoghue (7) and Meyers et al. (4) recommended repair of all torn ligaments and structures about the knee. Meyers et al. (4) showed good or excellent results in 13 of 16 knees with ligaments repaired, and good results in only one of 13 patients treated by manipulation and casting. In their review of 53 patients, they reported that 45 patients had ruptures of both the anterior and posterior cruciate ligaments.

Recommended Treatment Plan

We believe that accurate repair, appropriate rehabilitation, and patient cooperation are necessary if patients are to attain their best chance to return to athletic competition.

Frequently, a physician is available at the site when the athlete sustains an injury. If an immediate reduction can be performed, it is desirable. It is important for the person performing this immediate reduction to document the dislocation, however, and for this information to travel with the injured person to the emergency room. For example, if the knee redislocated or subluxed after a posterior dislocation injury had been reduced at the site, pressure would be placed directly on the popliteal artery, which in turn would create an untenable circulatory situation in the lower extremity.

If the patient arrives in the emergency room with the dislocation not reduced, reduction should be undertaken as soon as possible. After reduction, the distal arterial and neurologic examinations should be documented. If the foot is pulseless or if there is a question of adequate circulation below the knee, surgical intervention with arterial repair (or graft) should be done within 6 hr (Figures 10–3, 10–4). If an arteriogram would delay surgery beyond 6 hr after injury, the procedure should be omitted and surgical exploration should begin immediately. Anatomy of the popliteal vessels defines where the injury is. Fasciotomies should be done at the time of arterial repair. Repair of the ligamentous structures is not necessary at this time and can jeopardize the arterial repair or graft. Pins across the joint may be inserted at the time of arterial repair to retain the stability of the knee if necessary.

After arterial treatment, ligamentous repair can be carried out any time within the first 10–14 days without fear of jeopardizing the structures and their viability. Occasionally, a longer delay is required.

Dislocation should be considered in a severely traumatized knee which is reduced but shows marked multidirectional laxity with or without arterial injury. If there are no signs of arterial injury, surgery may be delayed until the facility, the surgeon, and the extremity are ready. Up to a 1-week delay may be needed for observation of circulatory status. During this time the knee can be kept in a flexed position (approximately 15°–30°), and a flexible movable cast brace can be applied. Just the small amount of motion available in a cast brace is desirable to encourage evacuation of fluids. No attempts should be made to perform vigorous quadriceps or hamstring strengthening exercises. The circulatory status of the extremity should be monitored at all times. During this period, treatment should include the straight leg raise, electrostimulation, short motions in the cast brace without motion applied with the hinges, application of ice, and constant elevation.

In most cases with severe ligamentous injuries about the knee, arthroscopy is contraindicated because of the capsular deficiency. Leakage of saline into the soft tissues could further inhibit the nutritional supply of the limb.

At the time of surgery, a systematic approach to all injured parts of the knee is undertaken through an anterior incision. This allows evaluation of the anterior and posterior cruciate ligaments plus the menisci, the patella, and its tendon. The joint surface should be thoroughly evaluated and the menisci assessed to determine if they can be repaired. If possible, repairs of the anterior and posterior cruciates are performed. There is generally enough laxity for these repairs to be made through the intercondylar notch. If not, the intercondylar notch can be widened laterally with an osteotome and curette to facilitate repair of the anterior cruciate ligament, and medially to allow repair of the posterior cruciate ligament (Figure 10–5). It is important to complete a bleeding bone hole for this repair.

We elect not to perform an intraarticular reconstruction of the anterior cruciate ligament in the multiply injured knee. The quality of the multiple repairs cannot be determined initially, and it is more appropriate to perform a reconstruction if the individual repairs are not satisfactory. In the repair of both the posterior cruciate and anterior cruciate ligaments, multiple sutures are used, with loop sutures placed through the ligament. This generally includes six absorbable sutures as well as six nonabsorbable sutures through the area which is incorporated into the bleeding bone bed. These sutures are then pulled through drill holes to the lateral intermuscular septum. *Initially, the sutures are not tied.* The posterior cruciate is repaired in the same fashion.

Next, we approach the posteromedial corner and medial collateral ligaments. These are appropriately repaired and oriented in their proper direction. It seems particularly important to orient the posterior oblique ligament in an anterior direction on its tibial attachment. AO/ASIF screws and barbed washers are used if necessary.

Then we approach the lateral side of the knee. An extraarticular reconstruction is performed utilizing the iliotibial band. This band is split longitudinally with a band width of approximately 1 cm. The band is split both anteriorly and posteriorly. Utilizing these splits, we can visualize the posterolateral corner of the knee. If damage is present in this area, as would be suspected, we fix this area with either multiple sutures or with a screw and washer to provide stability in the posterolateral corner. (This is the most commonly missed area of injury.) Then we address the lateral collateral ligament and repair appropriately. At this point, the joint is entered and the popliteal tendon identified. Generally, the tendon is ruptured and should be reattached to its initial area or advanced somewhat anteriorly. This can be done with either sutures or an AO/ASIF screw and washer.

The iliotibial band, which has previously been split, is fixed to an area 0.5 cm anterior to the lateral intermuscular septum and just proximal to the femoral condyle (the screw and washer are placed on a roughened femoral condylar surface). Utilizing first a 3.2 drill bit and then tapping the proximal side, we place a 6.5 cancellous screw under the band with a AO/ASIF barbed washer to fix the band in place. Then we place four interrupted nonabsorbable sutures through the lateral intermuscular septum and up into the band. This combination orients the band in two directions and eliminates both Lachman and anterior drawer signs. *Following this, the remainder of the ligaments are tied.* After the band sutures are applied, the band is divided proximal to the screw and washer, and the iliotibial tract is oversewn to recreate the iliotibial tract. If there is a question of patellar compression, lateral decompression is performed at the same time.

In the operating room, electrical stimulation is applied to the quadriceps and hamstring muscle groups. The limb is immobilized at 40°, and a cast brace is applied with no motion in the hinges of the cast brace initially.

In situations where motion and the return to activity are extremely important, the use of immediate constant passive motion has been used in a range of 40°–70° (Figure 10–6). We have managed only a few patients in this manner, and it is too soon to evaluate long-term benefits from the use of constant passive motion in our patients; neither has it been studied with large numbers of patients elsewhere. In the limited experience so far, passive motion has proved helpful in regaining motion early after the severe injury. Note that this motion is passive; early muscle pull across the joint could disrupt the repaired structures.

These patients will probably end up with some degree of laxity as the result of the severity of the injury. Grade 1 laxity is preferable, however, to the stiffness which frequently accompanies this type of injury.

If passive motion is not utilized, a cast brace is used with the knee position at about 40°. This is adjusted to a 40°–70° range that is continued throughout the treatment period. This range then is used for the first 8 weeks. The patient

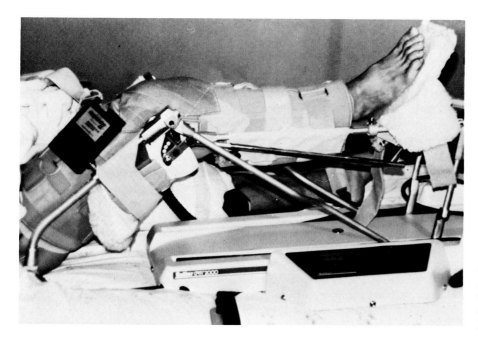

Figure 10-6 Knee dislocation after operation demonstrating the use of a cast brace, electrical stimulation, and continuous passive motion in a limited range of 40°–70°.

is allowed straight leg raises and quadriceps setting exercises in this position. After 8 weeks the brace is removed for exercise on the stationary bicycle and swimming. Patients may bear weight when "athletic," i.e., when the musculature about the knee is able to support the patient in a fluid manner.

The patient continues to use the brace in a 10°–90° range for 9–12 weeks and continues on an exercise program with muscle-strengthening exercises. The electrical stimulation is continued for 8 weeks and longer if there is some delay in regaining the quadriceps and hamstring muscle strength.

After bulk and strength about the knee are reestablished, the patient begins a series of proprioceptive exercises that include use of the tilt board and balance board (8). After this has been done, attention is directed to the person's regaining endurance and strength across the knee. Attempts at regaining this strength should be done in a range which does not significantly stretch the repaired structures, e.g., 45°–90° for quadriceps muscle exercises and whatever extension is available to 45° for hamstring exercise. After 6 months the range of motion can be increased for individual muscle groups. Exercises may be allowed which incorporate the contraction of both the hamstrings and the quadriceps at the same time.

Bicycling is the most appropriate athletic activity during the first 6 months. After 6 months, other exercises can begin. When running is begun, running upstairs is the most appropriate exercise, and this is incorporated into a "stadium stairs" running program. Downhill running is not recommended until 6–12 months after operation. Resumption of many activities depend on the patient's athletic ability. Participation in sports must be preceded by the person's regaining eccentric protection and proprioception.

Summary

The complications of knee dislocations may be disastrous and must be anticipated. In most series, a 25–30% incidence of arterial damage is reported. If the artery is not repaired, the incidence of amputation is high (up to 72.5%)

(2). The popliteal artery should be evaluated and vascular repair performed if needed. This must be completed within 6–8 hr after injury for optimal results. Peroneal nerve injuries are common, and permanent neurologic damage may result. The neurovascular injuries should be well documented at the time of injury and in the preinjury state. After all problems which affect limb survival are solved, open repair of all ligament injuries is recommended to provide ligamentous stability and congruity of the joint.

The surgeon performing the procedure must have a thorough knowledge of the anatomy of the knee. A thorough knowledge of appropriate rehabilitation techniques is equally important to guide the injured athlete through the immediate and late postoperative period.

REFERENCES

1. Debakey ME, Simeone FA (1946). Battle injuries of the arteries in World War II: an analysis of 2,471 cases. Ann Surg 123:534–579.
2. Green NE, Allen BL (1977). Vascular injuries associated with dislocation of the knee. J Bone Joint Surg 59A:236–239.
3. Kennedy JC (1963). Complete dislocation of the knee joint. J Bone Joint Surg 45A:889–904.
4. Meyers MH, Moore IT, Harvey JP (1975). Traumatic dislocation of the knee joint. J Bone Joint Surg 57A:430–433.
5. Mitchell JI (1930). Dislocation of the knee: report of 4 cases. J Bone Joint Surg 12:640–646.
6. Myles JW (1967). Seven cases of traumatic dislocation of the knee. Proc R Soc Med 60:279–281.
7. O'Donoghue DH (1955). An analysis of end result of surgical treatment of major injuries to the ligaments of the knee. J Bone Joint Surg 37A:1–13.
8. Steadman JR (1983). Rehabilitation of acute injuries of the anterior cruciate ligament. Clin Orthop 172:129–132.
9. Taylor AR, Arden GP, Rainey MA (1972). Traumatic dislocation of the knee: a report of 43 cases with special reference to conservative treatment. J Bone Joint Surg 54B:96–102.

Fixation of Tibial Shaft Fractures With Flexible Intramedullary Nails

11

Arsen M. Pankovich

Closed intramedullary nailing of tibial shaft fractures with rigid nails has been recommended and shown to be an effective method, particularly with simple oblique and transverse fractures of the tibial mid-shaft and segmental fractures (1,3,5,9,20). The main advantages of this method are good fixation of fracture fragments that allows early weight-bearing and virtually no infection. However, specialized skills and equipment and in some systems (e.g., the Kuntscher and AO nails) the need for preliminary reaming are disadvantages. Finally, only a short segment of the tibial mid-shaft is suitable for nailing.

Flexible intramedullary nails have been shown to be suitable for internal fixation of shaft fractures of the femur (6,14), tibia (11,15,17,19), and humerus (8). Nails are easily inserted, usually by a closed method, and require no preliminary reaming of the medullary canal. The method can be used in a variety of fracture types of the tibial shaft. Fixation is usually strong enough to allow for immediate weight-bearing without the use of cast immobilization while still preventing angulatory and rotational deformities.

Fracture Types

Tibial fractures are classified as undisplaced and displaced, the latter being usually unstable as well. For purposes of intramedullary nailing, tibial fractures can be classified in those which will be stable or remain unstable after nailing.

Stable Fracture Types

Transverse and short oblique fractures are stable after flexible nailing, and subsequent shortening and angulation will not occur. Early weight-bearing without a cast is a preferred postoperative regimen.

135

Fractures with unicortical comminution in which a single butterfly or a comminuted area involve less than one-half of the cortical circumference are stable after flexible nailing. If the area of the butterfly or comminution is larger than one-half of the cortical circumference, the fracture is potentially unstable and requires special handling to prevent angulatory deformities.

Unstable Fracture Types

In addition to the just described fracture with unicortical comminution, fractures with bicortical comminution are unstable after flexible nailing. In these fractures the greater part or the entire cortical circumference is comminuted. Shortening can occur after flexible nailing until the fibular fracture has healed.

Long oblique or spiral fractures are potentially unstable after flexible nailing because sliding of fragments can occur and result in shortening. Special handling of these fractures is also required.

When planning an intramedullary nailing procedure one should also look for linear, undisplaced, and often hardly visible fracture lines. These undisplaced fractures pose a problem in that they can become displaced during flexible nailing and convert a stable to an unstable fracture.

Operative Technique

In the majority of cases the procedure is done on a regular operating table adapted to allow for x-ray imaging by replacing the end of the regular table with a wooden hand table or a radiotransparent board. The image intensifier is easily positioned for anteroposterior viewing, and the leg is rotated for the lateral views. The knee is flexed to 30° over folded sheets for easier control of rotation of the extremity during insertion of the nails. A tourniquet can be used for intraoperative hemostasis but should be released before incisions are

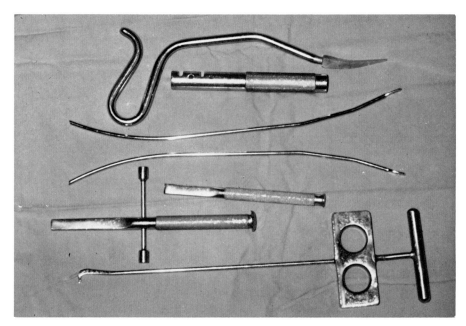

Figure 11-1 Instruments for flexible nailing (*top to bottom*): awl, bender, two flexible nails Ender C type, fine inserter, inserter, and extractor.

Tibial Shaft Fractures

closed. The leg is suitably draped free for easy manipulation during the procedure. A fracture table can be used for those cases of severe open fracture to facilitate debridement and when an ipsilateral femoral fracture exists that must be nailed.

The instruments are few and simple: impactor, fine impactor, awl, nail bender, and extractor (Figure 11–1). A drill and a 0.25-inch drill bit are needed to make portal holes. The nails are of two types: C and S nails. C-nails are used in the majority of cases. S-nails are sometimes used in comminuted fractures and when only one portal can be used.

Incisions are made from each side of the tibial tubercle obliquely to the level of the joint. The bone is then exposed bluntly. Portal drill holes are made: medially about 1.5–2 cm below the edge of the medial tibial plateau and laterally in Gerdy's tubercle. After the cortex is penetrated, the drill is oriented in the direction of the medullary canal. An awl is then used to enlarge the holes.

Proper nail length is determined using an image intensifier. The trial nail is placed on top of the leg with its eye at the level of a portal hole, and the fracture is reduced. The leading tip should reach the level of the tibial plafond. It is very important that the nails are long enough to engage the upper and lower metaphyses of the tibia close to the joint. In that way, they provide sufficient rotatory and bending stability and thus obviate the need for postoperative cast immobilization. Should a nail be too short or too long after it has been inserted, it should be replaced with another nail of proper length.

Nails are inserted simultaneously by two surgeons (Figure 11–2) or consecutively by one surgeon. They are driven to the fracture site, their position being checked with the image intensifier. It is of paramount importance now to reduce the fracture anatomically in order to prevent rotational and angular deformities, particularly internal rotation and posterior angulation while the nails are being driven down the medullary canal of the distal fragment.

When indicated, nailing can be done with the patient on a fracture table. The image intensifier must be positioned so that it can be rotated from the anteroposterior to the lateral position. If the knee can be flexed over an attach-

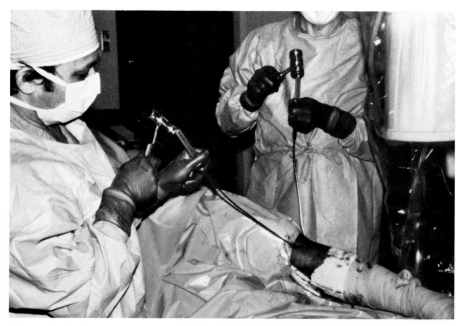

Figure 11–2 Insertion of the flexible nails is usually done simultaneously by two surgeons.

ment on the table, the procedure continues as described above. However, when the procedure is done without knee flexion support, it should be noted that there is a tendency for the thigh, and therefore the knee and the proximal fracture fragment, to fall in external rotation, thus leaving the distal fracture fragment and leg in the position of internal rotation. This will result in internal rotation malposition if not corrected. As the nails engage the distal fracture fragment, the thigh must be internally rotated. Only after that is done are nails driven down the distal fragment.

At the end of the procedure, a pressure dressing is applied over the incisions; rarely a posterior splint is used. The majority of patients need no cast immobilization because the fracture site is stable and only mild pain is present for 1–2 weeks. Patients are encouraged to ambulate with crutches and are allowed weight-bearing as tolerated, progressing to full weight-bearing as soon as possible. Usually the patient is ready to leave the hospital after 5–7 days.

Selection of Nails

It was recently demonstrated that flexible intramedullary nails maintain rotatory and angulatory alignment of fracture fragments, even though they allow rotation of fragments when a rotatory force is applied (7). Fragments then regain their original position when the force is released. Furthermore, it was shown that nails must be anchored in both the proximal and distal metaphyses

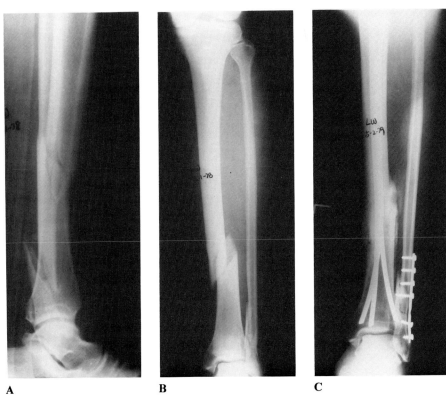

Figure 11–3 Short spiral fracture fixed with three flexible nails. **A** Lateral view. **B** Anteroposterior view. **C** Postoperative appearance: the fracture is solidly healed at 6 months.

An associated ankle fracture was also present. This was a comminuted supination-external rotation fracture of the fibula above the syndesmosis. Marked angulation of the distal fibular fragment was present. This fracture was plated after nailing of the tibial fracture. A short leg walking cast was used for 4 weeks.

of the tibia in order to provide stability, and therefore they must be long enough to do so. Nails 4.0 and 4.5 mm in diameter are available and should be used in tibial fractures. In most instances it is adequate to use only two 4.5-mm nails. If the medullary canal is wide, one more nail can be added. At least three 4.0-mm nails should always be used because they are more flexible. Only occasionally is the medullary canal too narrow to accept two 4.5-mm nails; however, in such a case the second nail can be a 4.0-mm nail or both nails can be of that diameter. It is my personal preference to use 4.5-mm nails because they are stronger, and in most cases only two nails are needed.

Indications, Pitfalls, and Possible Errors

The prime indication for fixation with flexible intramedullary nails is a short oblique or spiral fracture of the middle or distal third of the tibial shaft (Figure 11-3), which is often accompanied by a fibular fracture. This is a very unstable fracture which is difficult to reduce and to hold reduced in a cast. A transverse fracture of the tibia at the same level is also an excellent indication. Long oblique and spiral fractures can be successfully nailed, although they may have a tendency to slide and displace after the nailing if they are located in the proximal and distal third of the tibial shaft where the medullary canal widens and extends into the metaphyseal bone (Figure 11-4). This occurs if the nails

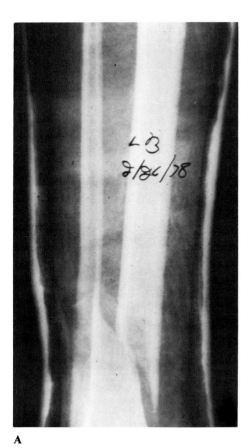
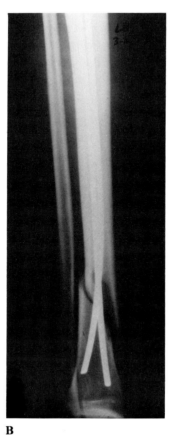
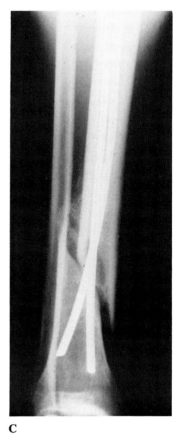

A   B   C

Figure 11-4 Sliding of fracture fragments after nailing. **A** Original film shows a long spiral fracture in the distal third of the tibial shaft. **B** Immediate postoperative film shows good reduction and alignment, although nails are short. **C** Film taken 6 weeks later shows sliding of the fracture fragments.

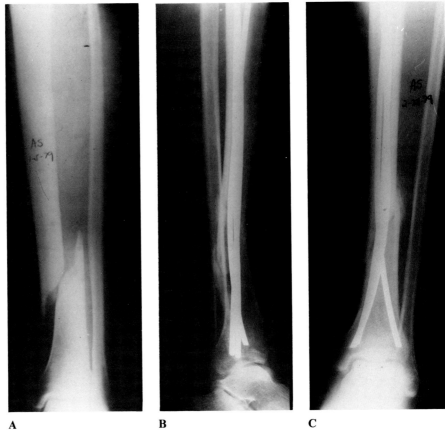

Figure 11–5 Appropriate nailing of a long spiral fracture of the tibia. **A** Original anteroposterior view. Lateral (**B**) and anteroposterior (**C**) views taken 8 weeks after nailing show the fracture to be healed in anatomic position. The nails have reached the tibial plafond and engage the metaphyseal bone.

are too short and do not engage the distal metaphysis sufficiently. Sliding can be prevented by making sure that the nails are long enough to penetrate well into the cancellous bone of the metaphysis and close to the tibial plafond. Whenever possible, nails should follow both the medial and lateral cortex of the distal fragment (Figure 11–5). Such fractures in the middle third of the shaft rarely slide and displace because the medullary canal is narrow in that area.

Oblique fractures in the upper third of the tibial shaft are sometimes difficult to nail and to keep reduced while being nailed. The Rush dictum of "V for victory and X for no good" should be kept in mind and is sometimes helpful (16). "V" indicates that the nail is inserted in the direction of the obliquity of the fracture: The direction of the fracture and the direction of the nail make a "V." The nail is therefore inserted from the side where the fracture line extends higher up on the cortex. When inserted from the opposite side, the nail is directed perpendicular to the fracture site, thus forming an "X." The nails also may have to be inserted into more centrally located portals in order to avoid penetration through the fracture site.

A fracture with unicortical comminution, particularly one with a large butterfly fragment, is quite suitable for flexible intramedullary nailing. Caution has to be taken to prevent a possible, though rare, angular deformity at the fracture site. This can happen during weight-bearing, particularly in a tall patient

Tibial Shaft Fractures

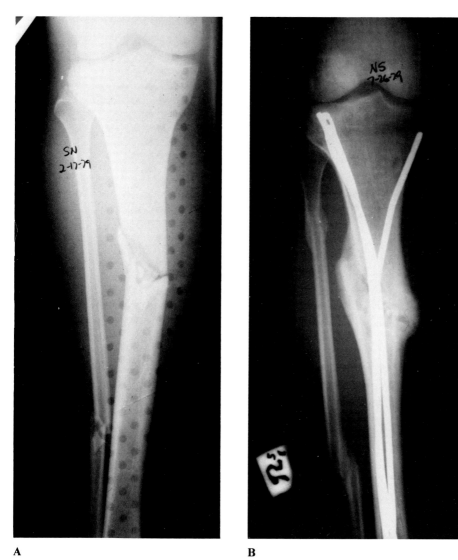

A   **B**

Figure 11-6 Tibial fracture with unicortical comminution. **A** Original anteroposterior film shows a tendency of the fracture for valgus angulation. **B** The fracture is healing in good alignment after fixation with three nails.

with long fracture fragments. An obvious way to avoid this problem is to insert more than two nails whenever possible (Figure 11-6).

Fractures with bicortical comminution may allow sliding of their fragments along the nails and produce significant shortening and angulation. Therefore the fracture must be protected in a long leg cast for 3-4 weeks, i.e., until there is initial fibrous healing of the tibial fracture and the fibula. This prevents shortening. Full weight-bearing is not allowed for 6-7 weeks.

Nailing of a fracture with bicortical comminution may be difficult because nails tend to penetrate outside the bone through the comminuted fracture site. In such cases the leading end of the nail should be straightened prior to insertion.

Problems may arise during the introduction of nails across the fracture site if undisplaced, linear, or hardly visible fractures are present, particularly at the base of bone spikes. These spikes may then be displaced if nails are driven vigorously across them. An oblique fracture may become a fracture with unicortical comminution and with a butterfly fragment, whereas the latter fracture may be converted to a fracture with bicortical comminution. If such undisplaced lines extend into the joint, a simple articular fracture may become a displaced one and require open fixation. To prevent these problems, it is important to look for extra fracture lines. The nails should be straightened with a bender at its leading curve so that less pressure is applied on the wall of the medullary canal and to the potential free fragments. Furthermore, pressure on these fragments can be avoided by turning away the tip of the nail when passing through such an area.

Segmental fractures are nailed in the same way as a singular fracture. If there is no comminution, fixation is usually strong enough to allow early unprotected weight-bearing.

Grades 1 and 2 open fractures can be nailed immediately after debridement and irrigation. It is easier to perform nailing initially than at a later date when the wound is healed and initial fibrosis at the fracture site makes the nailing much more difficult. My experience with grade 3 open fractures is limited. Extensive comminution is common in these fractures, and during insertion of nails undisplaced fragments may become displaced and make stable fixation impossible.

Ipsilateral fractures of the femur and tibia can be nailed simultaneously with the patient on a fracture table. After nailing the fractures, the leg compartments can be also released by fasciotomies if necessary.

Clinical Experience

In the personal series of 98 acute fractures in 95 patients treated at Cook County Hospital in Chicago and Kings County Hospital in Brooklyn, there were 76 closed fractures and 22 grade 1 and 2 open fractures. Four fractures were segmental, and three patients had bilateral tibial fractures. Three patients had ipsilateral tibial and femoral fractures; one required decompression of all leg compartments. The majority of fractures were in the distal third of the tibial shaft. At Cook County Hospital fractures were nailed using a fracture table, and those at Kings County Hospital were done on a regular operating table. Total anesthesia time was decreased when nailing was performed on a regular table. With few exceptions, an average procedure for closed nailing lasted 35–45 min. The average healing time was found to be 14 weeks, although in many cases the fracture was clinically healed in that the patient had little pain when ambulating unsupported.

Complications

In three cases nailing was attempted but not completed. In one case—a high tibial fracture with comminuted lateral wall of the proximal fragment—the lateral nails could not be inserted, and those from the medial portal always penetrated outside the bone before entering the distal fragment. In two other cases—also high tibial fractures—displacement of fracture fragments persisted after nailing, and the nails had to be removed.

In one case an 18° angular deformity developed and required renailing. Three additional patients had a 10° valgus angulation which was of no clinical significance.

Five tibias were nailed in rotational malposition. Two had internal rotation of 5° and one had 5° of external rotation, in each case of no clinical significance.

Tibial Shaft Fractures 143

Two tibias had more than 10° of internal rotation and required renailing in a correct position.

Osteomyelitis developed in two cases. In the first case a grade 3 open fracture with bicortical comminution was debrided and nailed 3 days after injury. Drainage was noted at 6 weeks and eventually required extensive debridement and open bone grafting after removal of the nails. In the second case a grade 2 open fracture was nailed 3 weeks after debridement and after the wound was healed. Ten days after nailing, drainage from the portals and the fracture site was noted and *Staphylococcus aureus* (coagulase-positive methicillin-resistant) was cultured. Protracted antibiotic treatment was required.

Shortening of the tibia was noted in four patients. In two cases, shortening of 0.5 and 1.0 cm was of no clinical significance. Shortening of 1.5 and 2.0 cm in two other cases was not acceptable, although the patients had no complaints.

Concluding Remarks

Flexible intramedullary nailing is a very suitable method for the treatment of tibial shaft fractures. It is applicable to a variety of fracture types and best for simple transverse and short oblique fractures, particularly in the middle and distal third of the tibial shaft. In these cases fixation is always stable and strong enough to allow early weight-bearing without the use of a cast. In other less-stable fracture types (e.g., fractures with unicortical and bicortical comminution) flexible intramedullary nails accomplish and maintain alignment of fracture fragments, although some of them may need short periods of immobilization in a cast. Fractures from about 8 cm below the tibial tubercle to about 7 cm above the tibial plafond are suitable for nailing.

In a great majority of cases, nailing is done as a closed procedure under control of an image intensifier. Only rarely does the fracture site have to be opened through a small incision in order to facilitate reduction of fracture fragments and for removal of the interposed soft tissues. Adjunctive fixation with cerclage wires, screws, or a plate, as in comminuted fractures of the femur (*13*), is essentially never necessary.

The method of flexible intramedullary nailing is easily learned because instrumentation is simple and the procedure does not require reaming of the medullary canal. After fixation of a fracture with flexible intramedullary nails, some motion still occurs at the fracture site and is sometimes referred to as controlled dynamic motion (*14*). This motion stimulates and promotes formation of external callus as was recently pointed out by McKibbin (*10*). This may explain a more consistent and earlier appearance of callus on roentgenograms and earlier clinical and roentgenographic evidence of bony union. Also, because reaming is not done, there is theoretically a greater preservation of the intramedullary blood supply.

It is well known that three significant complications may occur in the treatment of tibial shaft fractures: (a) nonunion and delayed union; (b) malposition and malunion; and (c) posttraumatic and postoperative osteomyelitis.

Nonunion has been reported at the rate of 0–10% by various authors using different methods (*2–4,9,11,12,17,18*). In the author's experience, one atrophic nonunion has occurred. Two cases of delayed union were also seen, both of which healed, although in one of them the nails were removed because it was thought that they were maintaining distraction of fracture fragments.

Malunion with 10° or more of valgus angulation was seen in three patients. This deformity, although of no clinical significance in these patients, could and should have been corrected at the time of nailing. Likewise, rotational malposition which required renailing could have been avoided. In all of these cases, surgical error resulted in malposition. However, in only one case did the increase in valgus angulation develop postoperatively and required renailing.

Osteomyelitis was seen in two cases. In the first case it probably developed because of a 3-day delay in debridement of a grade 3 open fracture. In the second case closed nailing was done 3 weeks after the injury in which a grade 2 open fracture was present. Osteomyelitis developed after the nailing.

In summary, it can be said that flexible intramedullary nailing of tibial shaft fractures is a method which provides good alignment of fracture fragments, allows for some motion at the fracture site and thus promotes external callus formation, uses nails that are easily inserted without exposure of the fracture site, allows early weight-bearing usually without cast immobilization, and causes few complications.

REFERENCES

1. Alms M (1962). Medullary nailing for fractures of the shaft of the tibia. J Bone Joint Surg 44B:328–339.
2. Anderson LD, Hutchins WC (1966). Fractures of the tibia and fibula treated with casts and transfixing pins. South Med J 59:1026–1032.
3. Bayne LG, Morris H, Wickstrom J (1960). Evaluation of intramedullary fixation of the tibia with the Lottes nail. South Med J 53:1429–1440.
4. Brown PW, Urban JG (1969). Early weight-bearing treatment of open fractures of the tibia: an end result study of sixty-three cases. J Bone Joint Surg 51A:59–75.
5. D'Aubigne RM, Maurer P, Zuchman J, Masses Y (1974). Blind intramedullary nailing for tibial fractures. Clin Orthop 105:267–275.
6. Eriksson E, Hovelius L (1979). Ender nailing in fractures of the diaphysis of the femur. J Bone Joint Surg 61A:1175–1181.
7. Haher TR, Devlin VJ, Freeman B (1983). Personal communication.
8. Hall RF Jr, Pankovich AM (1982). Closed flexible intramedullary nailing of humeral shaft fractures. Unpublished data.
9. Lottes JO (1974). Medullary nailing of the tibia with the triflange nail. Clin Orthop 105:253–266.
10. McKibbin B (1978). The biology of fracture healing in long bones. J Bone Joint Surg 60B:150–162.
11. Merianos P, Pazaridiss, Serenes P, et al. (1982). The use of Ender nails in tibial shaft fractures. Acta Orthop Scand 53:301–307.
12. Nicoll EA (1974). Closed and open management of tibial fractures. Clin Orthop 105:144–153.
13. Pankovich AM (1981). Adjunctive fixation in flexible intramedullary nailing of femoral fractures: a study of twenty-six cases. Clin Orthop 157:301–309.
14. Pankovich AM, Goldflies ML, Pearson RL (1979). Closed Ender nailing of femoral shaft fractures. J Bone Joint Surg 61A:222–232.
15. Pankovich AM, Tarabishy IE, Yelda S (1981). Flexible intramedullary nailing of tibial shaft fractures. Clin Orthop 160:185–195.
16. Rush LV (1976). Atlas of Rush Pin Technics, 2nd ed. Berivon Company, Miridian, Mississippi, pp. 88–98.
17. Saltzman M, Dobozi WR, Brash R (1982). Ender nailing of problem tibial-shaft fractures. Orthopaedics 5:1162–1171.
18. Sarmiento A (1967). A functional below-the-knee cast for tibial fractures. J Bone Joint Surg 49A:855–875.
19. Segal D (1982). Personal communication.
20. Zuchman J, Maurer P (1969). Two level fractures of the tibia: results in thirty-six cases treated by blind nailing. J Bone Joint Surg 51B:686–693.

External Fixation of Fibular Fractures

12

Richard A. Fischer
David Seligson

Fractures of the fibula can occur as isolated injuries from direct trauma, as part of the "tib-fib" fracture, and as a component of ankle fractures and pilon injuries. Certainly, most orthopaedists treat a closed bumper fracture nonoperatively and a fibular fracture in a pilon injury operatively. However, the exact indications for surgery in the great majority of fibular fractures are not as clear.

The clinical importance of the fibula to the normal articulating ankle joint has been stressed by Yablon (16) and others (9–11). The biomechanical basis for this fact was established by Greenwald (5), who demonstrated that the ankle joint has an 11–13 sq cm surface area for load-bearing. This is a larger articular surface than is found in the knee or hip, but the tolerance for joint discrepancy is lower. Breitenfelder in 1957 (1) and Willenegger in 1961 (15) demonstrated that widening of the ankle mortise secondary to small degrees of rotation and/or lateral displacement of the distal fibula diminishes the contact area in the tibiotalar joint. Ramsey (11) found that the tibiotalar contact area was reduced by 42% when the talus was displaced laterally by 1 mm. This reduction in surface area for load-bearing results in a concomitant rise in stress, thereby lowering the threshold for the subsequent development of arthrosis.

The ankle joint responds poorly to discrepancies in its anatomic configuration. Ankle fractures which result in incongruency of the normal articulation of the tibia, fibula, and talus lead to predictably poor results. Malka and Taillard (8) showed that nonoperative treatment of ankle fractures often leads to unsatisfactory results. Svend-Hansen et al. (14) in 1978 retrospectively studied 29 patients with unstable bi- or trimalleolar fractures with internal fixation of the medial malleolus alone. Fifty-five percent of these patients were classified as having unsatisfactory results or failure after only 4.8 years of follow-up.

Open reduction and internal fixation of fibular fractures about the ankle may effectively correct fibular length, rotation, and displacement irregularities. This form of treatment allows earlier mobilization of the ankle joint than does

145

immobilization in plaster without fibular fixation. Moreover, the indications for the operative restoration of fibular length, alignment, and rotation increase if the mortise is disrupted or the axis of the leg is disturbed.

Osteosynthesis of the fibula has come, for the most part, to mean screw or plate and screw fixation. By looking critically at our own patient material after fibular osteosynthesis, a stubborn incidence of swollen ankles, weepy wounds, and minor ulcers was apparent—the morbidity associated with rigid osteosynthesis of a subcutaneous bone. These complications arise in exchange for the complications of the "fracture disease" of nonoperative treatment and are underemphasized in a general enthusiasm for moving injured parts after surgery.

Those cases with marked soft tissue damage or preexisting poor tissue condition are precisely the ones where the greatest risks are present and for which another technique is needed. Does external fixation, as this other technique, provide an option for the management of fibular fractures; and if so, what are the relevant biomechanical considerations?

The fibula is not a static strut which serves as a source for muscle and ligament attachment. Studies have shown that the fibula rotates and translates with respect to the tibia in both an axial and a coronal plate (4,6,12). Therefore any device for achieving stability of distal fibular fractures must counter bending, axial compression and tension, shear, and rotational forces. Elastic fixation via external fixation can neutralize these forces. Burny (2,13) showed in a large series that elastic external fixation gives results comparable to other methods of closed and open fracture treatment for tibial shaft fractures. Furthermore, a small bone, e.g., the fibula, is even more conducive to elastic external fixation because of the smaller loads it must bear under normal conditions.

Lambert (7) demonstrated via strain gauge studies that one-sixth of the static load borne by the leg is carried by the fibula. Therefore in a static one-legged stance, the fibula of a 70-kg patient would transmit a load of slightly more than 11 kg. Eggshell touchdown or limited weight-bearing drastically reduces the force that the fibula would have to bear in the postoperative phase.

External fixation has the advantages of minimal soft tissue damage, adjustability, and removal. Internal fixation allows more precision in fracture reduction and repair of associated ligamentous injuries.

We have used external fixation of the fibula in the following situations: (a) Pilon fractures with crush or open injuries; (b) ankle fractures with crush or open injuries; (c) tibia shaft fractures with axial malalignment; (d) closed ankle and pilon fractures; (e) cases of polytrauma; and (f) ankle fractures with tibiofibula diastasis.

Method

Under spinal or general anesthesia the affected leg is prepared and draped free as a sterile field, and a roll is placed under the ipsilateral thigh. The fracture is visualized under fluoroscopic control with a mobile image intensifier. Biplanar x-ray control is achieved by either rotating the C-arm or manipulating the leg. Pin locations are determined using needle markers. Stab incisions are made, and 3-mm self-drilling Hoffmann half pins are inserted with the wimble. The pins are started by sharply striking with the T-wrench on the wimble to achieve cortical penetration. Pin spacing is determined visually. The pin groups are located to minimize the connecting rod length.

With short (Weber type A and B) distal fibular fractures a mini-Hoffmann can be used; with longer distal fragments (Weber C and shaft fractures) the

Fibular Fractures

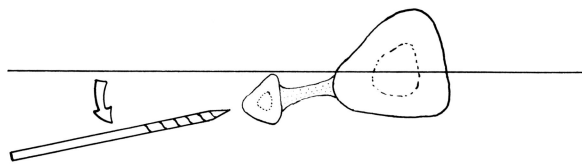

Figure 12-1 The fibula lies 16°-20° posterior to the coronal plane through the tibia (3,6).

C-series equipment is used. If significant damage to the syndesmosis is suspected or demonstrated under fluoroscopy, the pins are directed 20° anteriorly so intertibiofibular fixation is possible (Figure 12-1). The fracture is reduced manually by manipulating the leg and ankle and by applying direct pressure on the fracture fragments. A short connecting rod is placed, and the fixateur is blocked. The final position can generally be achieved after one or two trial reductions are checked with the image intensifier.

The tourniquet is then inflated, and fixation of associated tibial fractures may be performed. Permanent films confirm the reduction prior to leaving the operating room. The leg is placed in a plaster posterior splint, and the patient is nursed on a Bohler-Braun frame. At 48 hr postoperatively, a removable plastic posterior splint is substituted and active assisted range of motion therapy is initiated.

All patients are placed on intravenous cephazolin therapy during the preoperative and 48-hr postoperative period. As soon as intravenous antibiotics are stopped, the patient begins oral therapy with a broad-spectrum antibiotic (cephalexin or tetracycline) for as long as the fixateur is in place. Sutures, if present on the medial ankle, are removed at 2 weeks. At 4-6 weeks postoperatively eggshell touchdown weight-bearing is begun, and if a syndesmosis pin is present it is removed at 6 weeks in the office.

At 6-8 weeks postoperatively, weight-bearing is advanced as tolerated. The entire fixateur is removed without anesthesia in the office at 6-8 weeks. After fixateur removal, weight-bearing is advanced as tolerated.

Case Reports

Case I

O.M., a 20-year-old university sophomore on summer vacation was thrown from his motorcycle when he swerved to avoid a car backing out of a service entrance; he sustained a fracture of the right ankle and a laceration of the right knee. The ankle injury (Figure 12-2) consisted of a fracture of the medial malleolus and supramalleolar bending fibular fracture (PA III). There was also a deep abrasion on the anterolateral and lateral surfaces of the lower leg and ankle. The wounds were cleansed and dressed, and he was placed in calcaneal traction.

Six days after the injury the patient had closed reduction and external fixation of the fibula fracture under image intensification and an open reduction and internal fixation of the medial malleolus with two 4.0-mm cancellous screws (Figure 12-3). The fibula was percutaneously fixed with 3-mm half-pins which

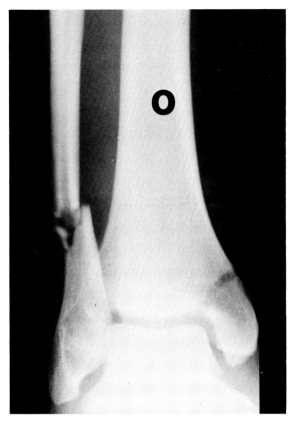

Figure 12–2 Case I. Preoperative view.

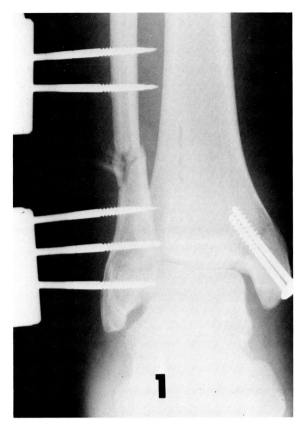

Figure 12–3 Case I. One week postoperatively.

were assembled into a Hoffmann C-series half-frame with a 5-mm connecting rod (Figure 12–4).

The patient returned to college and gradually was able to resume normal activity. He did not lose any time from classes. When he returned home for Thanksgiving recess, he had a full range of motion, walked without a limp, and had solid union of both fractures (Figure 12–5).

Eight months after the injury he was readmitted and the screws were removed from his medial malleolus (Figure 12–6). At 1 year after the injury the patient was at full vigorous activity without any signs of disability.

Case II

K.S. is a 37-year-old saleswoman who slipped on some ice in a driveway and fell, twisting her ankle in the process. She sustained a fracture of her ankle (PA III) (Figure 12–7). The injury was closed, and the neurovascular status of her left leg and foot was normal. She was placed in a posterior splint and nursed on a Bohler-Braun frame. On the first postinjury day, she underwent closed reduction and external fixation of the fibular fracture via a Hoffmann series C external fixateur and open reduction and tension band fixation of the medial malleolus.

After the external fixateur had stabilized the fibular fracture, a fifth half-pin was inserted across the fibula and into the tibia, serving as a syndesmosis pin. Tourniquet time for the entire procedure was 20 min (Figure 12–8). At 14 weeks postoperatively she was full weight-bearing with normal left ankle range of motion (Figure 12–9).

Fibular Fractures

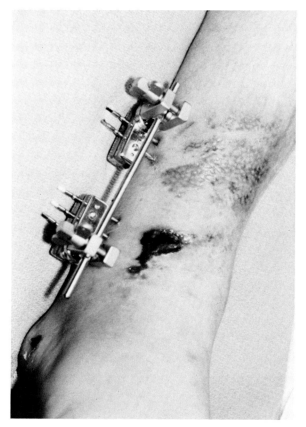

Figure 12–4 Case I. One week postoperatively.

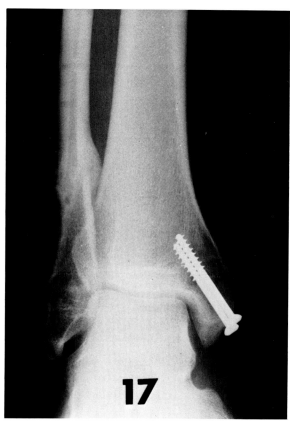

Figure 12–5 Case I. Seventeen weeks postoperatively.

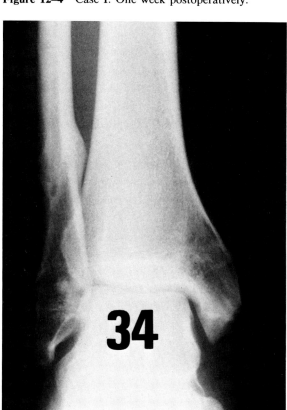

Figure 12–6 Case I. Thirty-four weeks postoperatively.

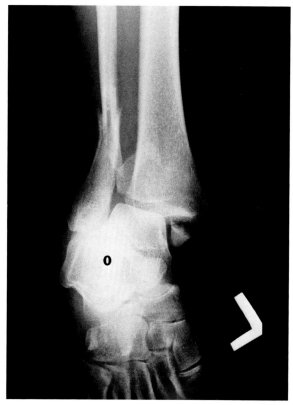

Figure 12–7 Case II. Preoperative view.

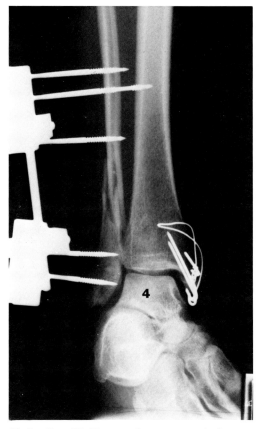

Figure 12–8 Case II. Four weeks postoperatively.

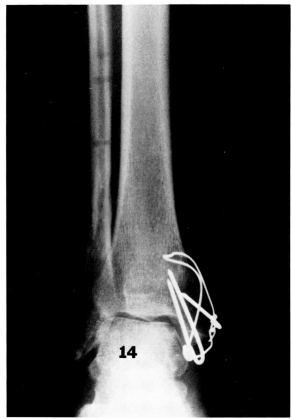

Figure 12–9 Case II. Fourteen weeks postoperatively.

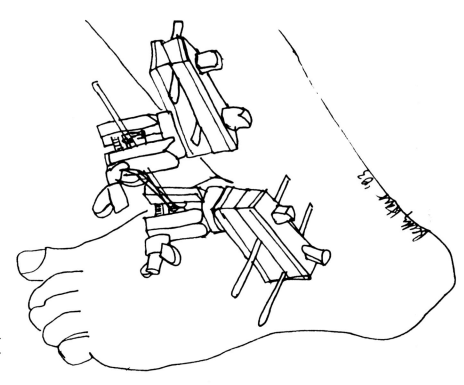

Figure 12–10 A patient's own interpretation.

Fibular Fractures

Conclusions

Patient acceptance of an external fixateur on the distal fibula is surprisingly high, as evidenced by a sketch by a proud wearer (Figure 12–10). The lack of a long lateral incision on the ankle is also appreciated.

External fixation can overcome the problems of rotational and length deformities in the fibula. The insertion of an additional pin into the tibia can solve problems associated with tibiofibular diastasis as well. The technique of elastic external fixation has been shown to be a successful option for treating certain fractures of the distal fibula. Encouragement with this technique has led us to consider the use of fixateurs more generally for these injuries.

REFERENCES

1. Breitenfelder H (1957). Der lange drehbruch des ausseren knochels (Verh Dtsch Orthop Ges Beiheft). Z Orthop 88:33–36.
2. Burny F (1982). Elastic external fixation. In: Concepts in External Fixation, edited by Seligson D, Pope MH. Grune & Stratton, New York, pp. 67–68.
3. Caillet R (1977). Foot and Ankle Pain. Davis, Philadelphia.
4. Close R (1956). Some applications of the functional anatomy of the ankle joint. J Bone Joint Surg 38A:761–781.
5. Greenwald S (1977). Cited by Stauffer RN, Chao EYS, Brewster RC: Force and motion analysis of the normal diseased and prosthetic ankle joint. Clin Orthop 127:189.
6. Kapandji IA (1970). The Physiology of the Joints, Vol. 2: Lower Limb. Churchill Livingstone, Edinburgh.
7. Lambert LL (1971). The weight-bearing function of the fibula: a strain gauge study. J Bone Joint Surg 53A:507.
8. Malka JS, Taillard W (1969). Results of nonoperative and operative treatment of fractures of the ankle. Clin Orthop 67:159–168.
9. Mathieu MP (1936). Reconstruction de la mortaise tibio-peroniere dans le traitement des fractures malleolaires. Livre jubilaire offert au Lambotte. Vromant and Co. Imprimataeurs diteurs, Bruxelles, pp. 315–322.
10. Mitchell WG, Shaftan GW, Sclafani SJA (1971). Mandatory open reduction: its role in displaced ankle fractures. J Trauma 19:602–615.
11. Ramsey PL, Hamilton W (1976). Changes in tibiotalar area of contact caused by lateral talar shift. J Bone Joint Surg 58A:356–357.
12. Scranton PE, McMaster JH, Kelly E (1976). Dynamic fibular function: a new concept. Clin Orthop 118:76–81.
13. Seligson D, Pope MH (1982). Concepts in External Fixation. Grune & Stratton, New York.
14. Svend-Hansen H, Bremerskov V, Baekgaard N (1978). Ankle fractures treated by fixation of the medial malleolus alone: late results in 29 patients. Acta Orthop Scand 49:211–214.
15. Willenegger H (1961). Die behandlung der luxations-frakturen des oberen sprunggelenkes nach biomechanische gesichtspunkten. Helv Chir Acta 28:225–239.
16. Yablon IG (1979). Ankle fractures—internal fixation. AAOS Instructional Course Lectures 28:72–93.

Triplane Fractures of the Distal Tibial Epiphysis

13

Phillip G. Spiegel
Jeffrey W. Mast
Daniel R. Cooperman
Gerald S. Laros

The purpose of this chapter is to update and add to our knowledge of triplane fractures of the distal tibial epiphysis.

Historical Review

Prior to the article by Cooperman et al. (*1*), a few authors throughout the years (*9,11,13,18,21*) had described fractures now popularly called triplane fractures. Since that time many others (*2,3,6,7,15,20*) have contributed to our understanding of this interesting and complex fracture of the adolescent distal tibial epiphysis.

Definition and Anatomy

The fracture is defined as an injury to the distal tibial epiphysis in which the fracture plane has sagittal, transverse, or horizontal, as well as coronal or frontal, components with fracture lines in the metaphysis, physis, epiphysis, and into the ankle joint. Roentgenographically, on plain films it most commonly has the appearance of a Salter-Harris type III fracture on the anteroposterior view and a Salter-Harris type II or IV fracture on the lateral view. Occasionally the posterior metaphyseal fracture is also seen on the anteroposterior view (Figure 13–1). Based on plain x-rays, tomography, computed tomography (CT) scans, and/or operative findings, the injury may consist of two, three, or four fragments. Various anatomic configurations of Salter-Harris type II, III, and IV lesions are also seen when utilizing these diagnostic modalities.

Marmor's description of the anatomy of the fracture (*13*) was based on operative findings of three fragments: (a) the tibial shaft; (b) the anterolateral

153

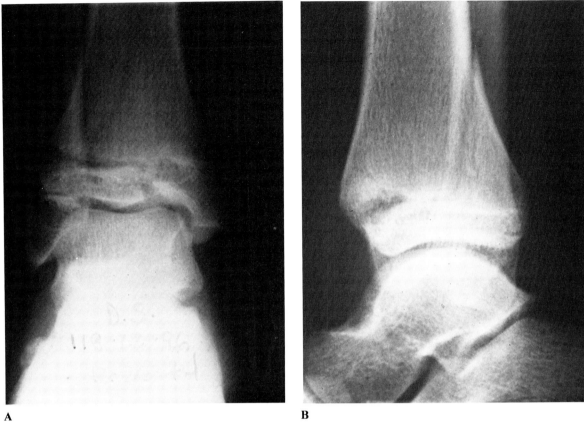

Figure 13–1 Common triplane fracture configuration. **A** A Salter-Harris type III lesion is seen as is the posterior metaphyseal fracture.

Figure 13–1B A Salter-Harris type II fracture is identified. There is no anterior displacement of any epiphyseal fragments.

epiphyseal fragment; and (c) the remainder of the epiphysis medially and posteriorly, attached to the posterior metaphyseal piece and the fibula (Figure 13-2). If seen alone, the free anterolateral piece mimics the juvenile Tillaux fracture (discussed under the differential diagnosis).

Lynn (*11*) described two cases, one of which was probably a three-fragment fracture, and gave the name "triplane fracture" to this entity. Torg and Ruggiero (*21*) operated on a similar fracture thought to be three fragments.

Cooperman et al. (*1*) studied five of 15 triplane fractures by anteroposterior and lateral tomograms and found a two-fragment fracture in those five patients. One fragment consisted of the fibula, the attached posterior metaphyseal piece, and the lateral and posterior medial portion of the epiphysis. The second fragment consisted of the tibial shaft and attached medial malleolus and the remaining anteromedial portion of the epiphysis (Figure 13-3). On anteroposterior (AP) tomograms, the sagittal Salter-Harris type III fracture is seen in the anterior cuts but is lost posteriorly. This finding on the AP tomograms is consistent with either a two- or three-fragment fracture configuration as the posterior metaphyseal-epiphyseal part of the fracture remains as one piece in all triplane fractures (Figure 13-4B–E). If the tibial shaft and medial malleolus appear to remain in continuity anteriorly and the anterolateral epiphyseal fragment appears to be in continuity with the posterior metaphysis, a two-fragment fracture is

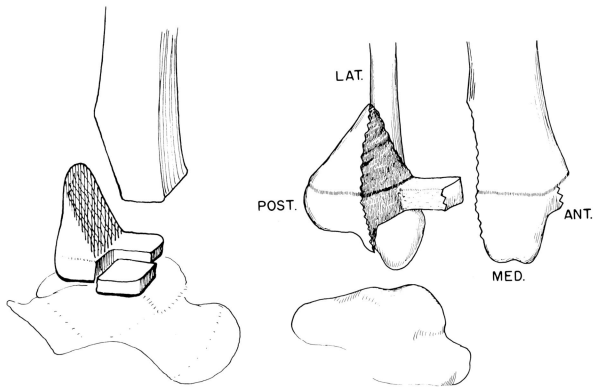

Figure 13-2 Three-fragment Marmor triplane fracture, showing the tibial shaft, the free anterolateral piece, and the remainder of the epiphysis, metaphysis, and fibula as a third piece. From Rang (18).

Figure 13-3 Two-fragment triplane fracture with the tibial shaft and medial malleous and anteromedial portion of the epiphysis as one fragment. The second fragment consists of the remainder of the metaphysis, epiphysis, and attached fibula. From Cooperman et al. (1).

more likely (Figure 13-5A). If on anteroposterior tomograms the tibial shaft does not appear to be in continuity with the medial malleolus anteriorly and the anterolateral tibial epiphyseal piece appears to be free, a three-fragment fracture is more likely. The distinction between two- and three-fragment fractures, however, is best made from lateral tomographic cuts. From laterally to medially, in a two-part triplane fracture the appearance of a Salter-Harris type II fracture is seen laterally and the Salter-Harris type IV fracture is seen medially. This indicates that the lateral epiphyseal and posterior metaphyseal-epiphyseal fragment piece and fibula are one unit (i.e., a free anterolateral piece is not present). Medially, the fracture line extends from the metaphysis through the growth plate and epiphysis (Salter-Harris type IV), indicating the separation of tibial shaft-medial malleolus and anteromedial portion of the epiphysis as the second fragment (Figures 13-5B and 13-9A, below). A CT scan of a two-fragment fracture confirms this configuration and corroborates the findings of Karrholm et al. (6) (Figure 13-6).

In a three-part Marmor fracture, on lateral tomograms the reverse picture would be true. The Salter-Harris type IV fracture would be seen laterally through the metaphysis, growth plate, and epiphysis as the anterolateral epiphyseal piece separates from the rest of the epiphysis. The Salter-Harris type II lesion would be evident more medially as the posterior-metaphyseal and medial-epiphyseal piece, and the fibula would be a second unit, with the tibial shaft as a third unit. Additionally, the free anterolateral epiphyseal piece, if displaced, should

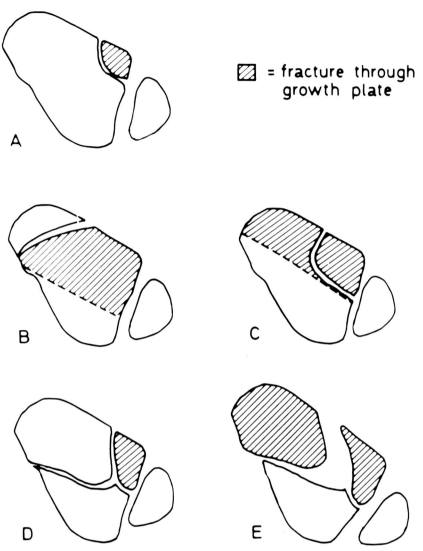

Figure 13-4 Five cases which show the epiphyseal fracture in different intraarticular supination-eversion injuries. Section through the growth plate. *Shaded area:* fracture through the growth plate. *White area:* solid connection between the epiphysis and metaphysis. **A** Tillaux fracture, two-fragment type. **B** Triplane fracture, two-fragment type. **C** Triplane fracture, three-fragment type according to Marmor (13), Torg and Ruggiero (21), and Rang (18). **D** Triplane fracture, three-fragment type according to Gerner-Schmidt. **E** Triplane fracture, four-fragment type. From Karrholm et al. (6).

appear anteriorly on the lateral tomograms in contrast to a two-fragment triplane fracture. Speculatively, in a Marmor-type three-part fracture, the medial malleolus is not a part of the tibial shaft and would not be contiguous with it on lateral tomograms, as is the case with two-fragment fractures. Such a three-fragment fracture constitutes a Salter-Harris type II, III, and IV injury (6). Peiro et al.'s (16) one case of a three-fragment fracture (the other five cases being two-fragment fractures) was diagnosed by tomograms and consisted of: (a) a free anteromedial epiphyseal fragment with the medial malleolus; (b) an anterolateral epiphyseal fragment and attached posterometaphyseal fragment

Distal Tibial Epiphysis Fractures

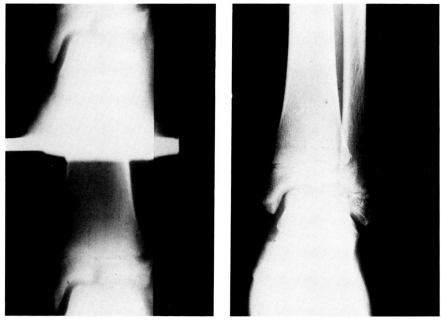

Figure 13–5 Tomograms of a patient with a two-fragment fracture. **A** Anteroposterior view with a plain film on the right and tomographic cuts on the left. Cuts show a probably intact medial malleolus and tibial shaft, but there is difficulty in evaluating the anterolateral epiphyseal piece.

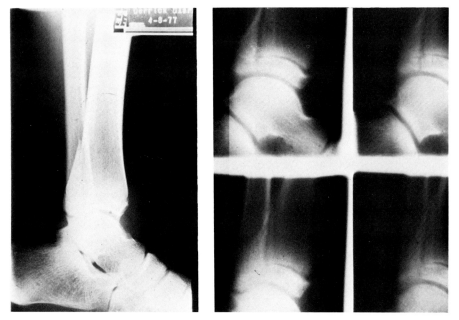

Figure 13–5B Lateral tomograms with a plain film on the left and tomographic cuts going laterally in a counterclockwise fashion on the right. Note the Salter-Harris type IV injury medially and the Salter-Harris type II injury laterally with an intact anterolateral epiphyseal piece.

and fibula; and (c) the tibial shaft (Figure 13–7). This case represents a variant because the free piece was not an anterolateral but an anteromedial fragment. (Karrholm's case 5, seen in Figure 13–4E, also has a free anteromedial fragment.) It seems that in most three-fragment fractures the third piece, the tibial shaft,

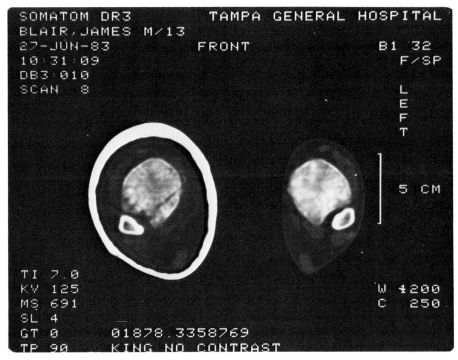

Figure 13–6 CT scans of a patient with a two-fragment triplane fracture. The fractured extremity has a cast on, which is seen at the left of the scan. The legs are somewhat externally rotated, and the cuts are 3–4 mm apart, going proximally to distally. **A** Note the posterior metaphyseal coronal fracture.

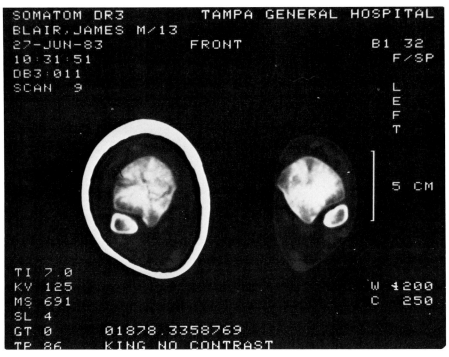

Figure 13–6B Extension of this fracture, medially to laterally.

Distal Tibial Epiphysis Fractures

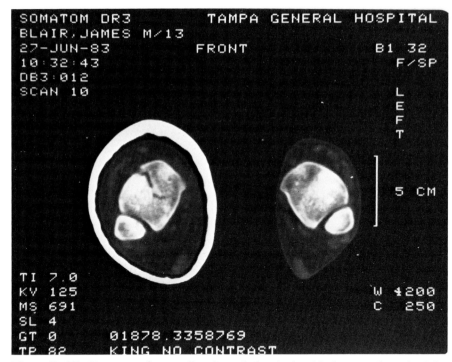

Figure 13–6C Transverse fracture line through the physis with the anterolateral epiphyseal piece intact. The tibial shaft and medial malleolus are beginning to separate (corresponds roughly to Figure 13–4B).

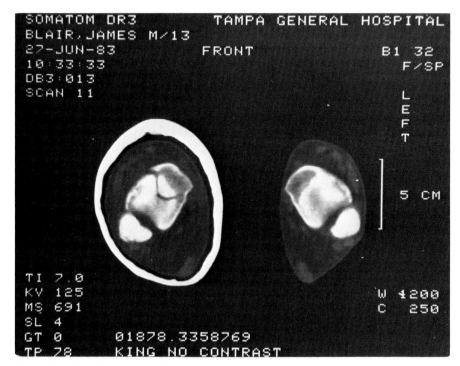

Figure 13–6D The tibial shaft and medial malleolus are one piece. The posterior metaphysis and the remainder of the epiphysis have remained intact in all cuts. (Case courtesy of Ortelio Rodriguez, M.D., Tampa, Florida.)

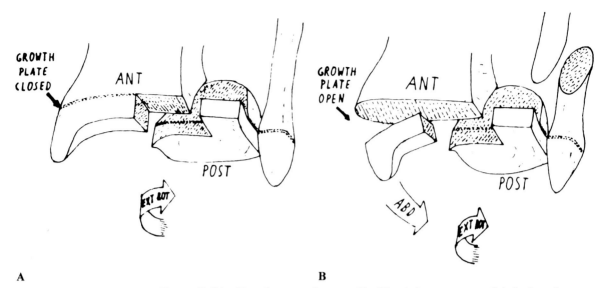

Figure 13–7A Two-fragment fracture. **B** Piero's interpretaton of their three-fragment fracture including fractures of the medial malleolus and fibula. From Peiro and Aracil (16).

does not carry with it any portion of the tibial epiphysis, perhaps indicating that these fractures with more pieces occur in younger patients with as yet unfused or fusing distal tibial epiphyses and a higher level of energy injury. An exception to this might be the fracture described in Figure 13–4D, a triplane injury attributed to Gerner-Smidt by Karrholm et al. (6) that was composed of three fragments: (a) an anterolateral part of the epiphysis separated from the metaphysis (as in a Marmor triplane); (b) a posterior metaphyseal fragment with the posterior part of the epiphysis attached to it (as with all triplanes); and (c) an anteromedial fragment consisting of the rest of the epiphysis attached to the metaphysis (as the tibial shaft fragment in a two-fragment fracture).

Denton and Fischer (2) further added to the literature by describing a two-fragment "medial triplane fracture." They referred to the configurations of Marmor (13) (three-part fracture) and Cooperman (1) (two-part fracture) as "lateral triplane fractures." Their medial triplane fracture on tomograms consisted of: (a) an anterolateral epiphyseal fragment which remains intact and attached to the tibial shaft and fibula; and (b) a medial and posterior epiphyseal fragment which is displaced medially and posteriorly along with a small portion of the posterior metaphysis (Figure 13–8). On plain x-rays, a Salter-Harris type IV lesion is seen in the lateral view as a large coronal or frontal portion of the epiphysis in contrast to the "lateral triplane." Additionally on the lateral view, the posterior metaphyseal spike is very short. Finally, a larger portion of articular surface is involved in the medial triplane (approximately 60%) as opposed to the lateral triplane (approximately 25%).

Although lateral tomograms might show a Salter-Harris type II lesion medially and a type IV lesion laterally, in both the two-fragment medial triplane and the three-part Marmor lateral triplane fractures the differences in width of the remaining anteromedial epiphysis (small in the medial triplane fracture), the height of the posterior metaphyseal fragment (short in medial triplane), and the displacement of the third piece—the tibial shaft with an epiphyseal fragment in the medial triplane—should be sufficient to make the two fractures discernible. A two-part lateral triplane fracture again shows a Salter-Harris type IV lesion medially and a Salter-Harris type II lesion laterally, making it

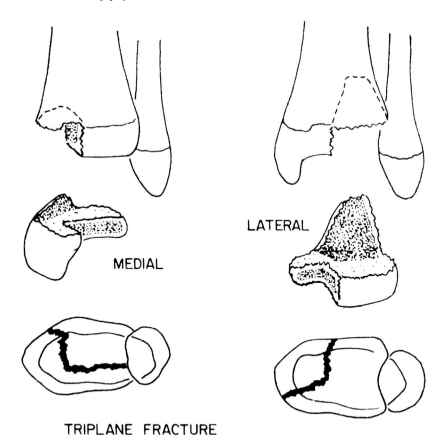

Figure 13–8 Two-fragment medial triplane fracture (*left*) and two-fragment lateral triplane fracture (*right*). From Ogden (15).

distinctive from either the two-part medial or the three-part lateral Marmor triplane fracture. Therefore the questions to be answered on the lateral tomograms are:

1. How many fragments are there (based on the location of the coronal fractures)?
2. Is the posterior metaphyseal spike in continuity with the anteromedial epiphysis and malleolus (medial triplane, three-part Marmor lateral triplane) or the lateral epiphysis (Cooperman two-part lateral triplane; Peiro three-fragment triplane)?
3. Is the tibial shaft free (three-part Marmor lateral triplane, three-part Peiro triplane) or in continuity with the medial malleolus (two-part Cooperman lateral triplane) or with the anterolateral epiphyseal fragment and fibula (two-part medial triplane)?

Dias and Giegerich (3) investigated eight triplane injuries, six of which were three-fragment fractures. The width of the fragment comprising the anterolateral epiphyseal piece was 40–50% of the width of the epiphysis, and the fragment was laterally displaced 1–4 mm. The posterior metaphyseal spike was 1–4 cm in height with 0–4 mm posterior displacement. When present, the fibular fracture was located 4–6 cm proximal to the tip of the lateral malleolus and usually ran obliquely from posterosuperior to anteroinferior. Karrholm et al. (7) believed that the fibular fracture is a long spiral, starting distally and close to the growth plate medially, and then runs laterally and posteriorly as it exits proximally. In Dias and Giegerich's series (3), both two-fragment triplane fractures had no associated fibula fracture.

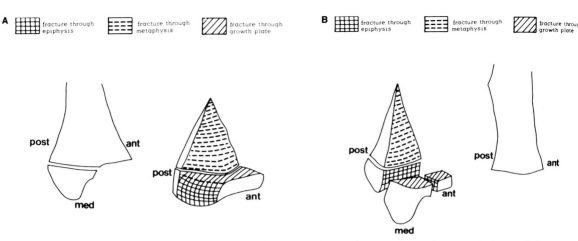

Figure 13–9 **A** Two-fragment triplane fracture. Note the curved shape of the growth plate and epiphyseal fracture (see Figure 13–4B). **B** Four-fragment triplane fracture (see Figure 13–4E). From Karrholm et al. (6).

By far the most extensive work to date on children's ankle fractures, including triplane injuries, is by Karrholm and his associates (6–8). Their classification is both anatomic and traumatologic, including the use of computed tomography in four cases of triplane fractures (Figure 13–4B–E). They found that triplane fractures consisted of two to four fragments, representing three-fracture patterns, and conventional x-rays could not differ between the two- and three-fragment fractures. They believed that the CT scan registered the epiphyseal and metaphyseal fractures in detail including the exact displacement of the fragments. Given that, one case with a three-fragment fracture as diagnosed by tomograms and CT scan was found to have a fourth fracture, a nondisplaced anteromedial part of the growth plate. Using tomography and CT scans, the epiphyseal fracture in the two-fragment triplane started more medially and had a transverse or curved shape to it as opposed to the three-fragment type, which started more laterally and had a more perpendicular course. They also found that the metaphyseal fragment was always posterior or dorsal, with the apex located posteromedially, straight posteriorly, or sometimes posterolaterally (Figure 13–9).

Growth Plate Maturation

Kleiger and Mankin (9) examined anteroposterior roentgenograms of the ankles in 60 persons between the ages of 12 and 20. In 24 of these ankles the epiphyseal plate showed an elevation or hump about 1 cm from its medial margin. They believed that this hump might prevent displacement of the medial portion of the epiphysis when lateral rotation stress was applied. In 22 ankles closure of the epiphyseal plate had already started, and their roentgenograms suggested that fusion of the distal tibial epiphysis proceeds in an irregular manner. It seemed to close first in the middle portion, then on the medial side, and lastly in the lateral portion, with the entire process taking about 18 months. Closure appears to first take place posteriorly rather than anteriorly, as evidenced by the posterior metaphyseal piece and epiphysis remaining as a unit no matter what type of triplane fracture is identified (Figure 13–10). Closure is usually complete by 14 years of age but it can vary, closing earlier in girls than boys and sometimes not closing until age 18.

Distal Tibial Epiphysis Fractures

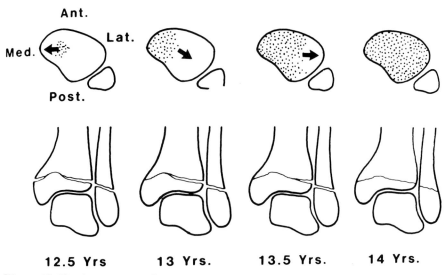

Figure 13–10 Average age of onset and normal fusion pattern in the distal tibial epiphysis. From MacNealy et al. (12).

Mechanism of Injury

Karrholm et al. (7) classified triplane fractures as supination-eversion injuries, utilizing a traumatologic classification developed experimentally by Gerner-Smidt for children with open growth plates. Gerner-Smidt produced ankle fractures of the supination-eversion type in children older than age 10 years and spiral fractures of the tibia in children under age 7 years. This indicates that one mechanism of injury can be responsible for different fracture patterns depending on the previously described skeletal maturity of the distal tibial epiphysis. By definition, all supination-eversion injuries have a posterior metaphyseal spike. Karrholm et al. divided their series of intraarticular fractures of the distal tibia into four stages: The juvenile Tillaux fracture comprised stages I and II; stage III is a triplane fracture without a fibula fracture (two, three or four fragments); and stage IV is a triplane fracture (two, three, or four fragments) with a fibula fracture (Figure 13–11). The reader should consult their detailed paper for further analysis and breakdown of the categories (7). Dias and Tachdijan (4) modified Lauge-Hansen's studies utilizing the position of the foot at the time of trauma and the direction of the abnormal force. They believed, as does Karrholm, that the juvenile Tillaux fracture is produced by the same mechanism of injury that produces the triplane fracture. They noted that the triplane fracture is probably produced by a "combination of external rotation and plantar flexion forces." In a later paper, Dias and Giegerich (3) noted that both the juvenile Tillaux and the triplane fracture mechanism of injury are "pure external rotation of the foot without either pronation and supination." A grade I injury (also as per Karrholm et al.) produces the isolated Salter-Harris type III juvenile Tillaux fracture of the anterolateral corner of the epiphysis. Further external rotation then produces a triplane fracture (three fragments), and lastly extreme external rotation results in the additional spiral fibula fracture. Cooperman et al. (1) postulated that an axial external rotation load on a plantar flexed foot produces a triplane fracture. They based their theory on their studies of children's ankle fractures, particularly Salter-Harris type II injuries (19). They divided

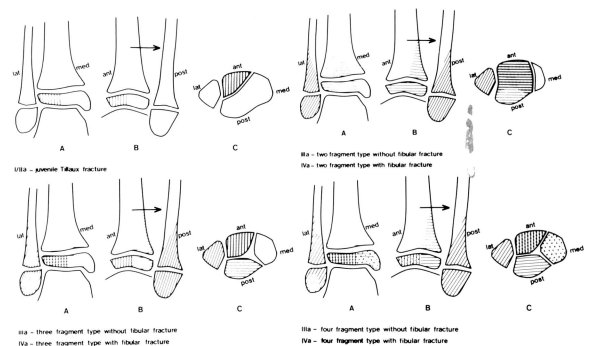

Figure 13–11 Stages of supination-eversion injuries in children with open growth plates and intraarticular distal tibial fractures. **A** Anteroposterior view. **B** Lateral view. The fibula is illustrated to the right of the tibia. **C** Section through the growth plate of the distal tibia and the fibula, respectively. From Karrholm et al. (6). ||||| different fracture, ≡ fragments of, ░░ distal tibia, different fracture, //// fragments of, distal fibula, separation through   growth plate of distal tibia and/or fibula.

that group into proposed mechanisms of injury—abduction, plantar flexion, rotational, and unclassified—and found that the plantar flexion and rotational radiologic fracture patterns resembled the triplane fracture patterns but in an unfused distal tibial physis. It was theorized that the intraarticular tibial portion of the fracture was not produced because the biomechanical immaturity of the growth plate did not allow a fulcrum to lever against during the injury.

In summary, all authors agree that at least one (and perhaps the most important) component of the mechanism of injury in triplane fractures is external rotation. Whether the foot is supinated, plantar flexed, axially loaded, or combinations thereof at the time of injury may account for the various fracture patterns seen. This again depends on the maturity of the distal tibial growth plate at the time of injury.

Diagnosis

Each of the three fractures included in the differential diagnosis of a triplane injury occurred in patients with an average age greater than 13.5 years in the University of Chicago series (*19*). The radiologic differential diagnosis of a triplane fracture includes:

1. A Salter-Harris type III injury seen only on the AP view with a more centrally or laterally placed sagittal fracture line than the usual supination-inversion injury of the medial malleolus. On the lateral x-ray or lateral tomograms there is a complete absence of a fracture line (Figure 13–12A,B). This

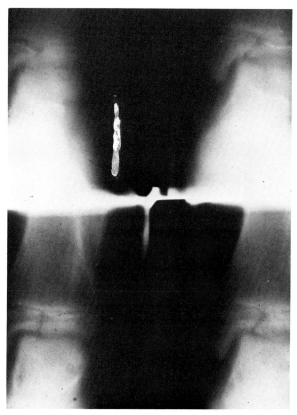 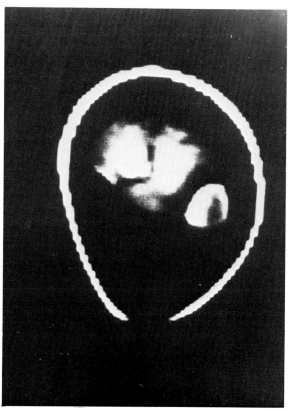

Figure 13–12A Anteroposterior tomographic cuts of a central Salter-Harris type III injury of the distal tibial epiphysis. No fracture line was seen on lateral tomographic views.

Figure 13–12B CT scan of the same fracture showing the fracture line to be entirely sagittal with no coronal component. Note that the fracture line extends posteriorly through the entire epiphysis.

Salter-Harris "central type III" injury was present in six of the 49 Salter-Harris type III fractures in the University of Chicago series (*19*).

2. A juvenile Tillaux fracture is defined as a Salter-Harris type III injury of the anterolateral part of the tibial epiphysis (Figure 13–13). Radiologically, the fracture is seen on the mortise view when the fibula is not superimposed on the lesion (Figure 13–14A). Anterior displacement of the piece may be seen on the lateral view (Figure 13–14B). There are no other associated fracture lines seen in the metaphysics on the lateral view as there would be in a three-part Marmor lateral triplane. However, MacNealy et al. (*12*) described six of their 27 cases of juvenile Tillaux fracture that did have a posterior malleolar fracture seen on the lateral view but were not triplane fractures. They believed that this was a combination which has not been previously described. Rang (*18*), Dias and Giegerich (*3*), and Karrholm et al. (*7*) suggested that the juvenile Tillaux fracture is an avulsion fracture caused by external rotation of the foot acting on an intact anterior inferior tibiofibular ligament attached to the as yet unfused anterolateral tibial epiphysis. Ogden (*15*) suggested that because the foot is externally rotated the talus applies a compression-torque stress that propagates a crack through the articular surface up to the growth plate, which then fails in shear.

Further discussions of this fracture with reference to treatment and prognosis are found in recent articles by Dingeman and Shaver (*5*), Letts (*10*), Mac-Nealy et al. (*12*), Molster et al. (*14*), and Protas and Kornblatt (*17*). Kleiger and Mankin's (*9*) paper contains the most detailed description of this injury.

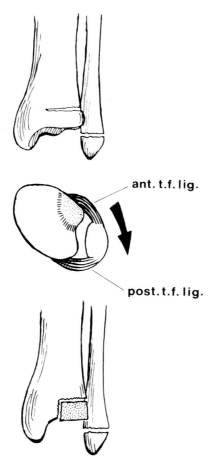

Figure 13–13 Juvenile Tillaux fracture and proposed mechanism of injury. From Rang (18).

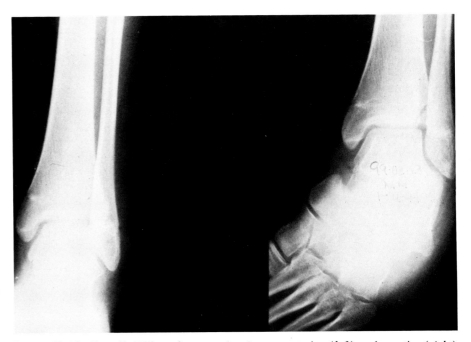

Figure 13–14 Juvenile Tillaux fracture. **A** Anteroposterior (*left*) and mortise (*right*) view. The mortise view gives the best representation of the fracture.

Treatment

Closed treatment remains the initial option for the vast majority of triplane fractures. Tinnemans and Severijnen (20) reviewed the literature up to 1979 and found that seven of 35 (20%) triplane fractures were treated by operative means. In contrast, Dias and Griegerich (3) operated on three of their six three-part fractures and treated their two two-part fractures with closed reductions. The patients operated on were younger in age with open tibial physes. Two of these patients had fibula fractures, again indicating that a more severe injury producing a multifragmented triplane fracture occurs in a young patient with a less mature tibial physis. It may be this type of triplane fracture that most often needs an open reduction. In those three cases, closed reduction failed, with more than 2 mm residual displacement present. Their closed treatment consisted of internal rotation of the foot with forward traction on the heel and maintenance of the position for 6 weeks in a long leg cast. Their operative treatment consisted of no fibular fixation with anteromedial and anterolateral incisions for direct visualization and reduction of the tibial fragments. Internal fixation devices are not mentioned nor were operative x-rays shown in their paper.

Denton and Fischer's (2) medial triplane was operated on through a medial approach. Fixation was accomplished with two smooth Kirschner wires which were removed 6 weeks after operation. There was no weight-bearing for 3 months total time.

Karrholm et al. (7) had three cases that could be treated satisfactorily by closed reduction and seven cases where closed reduction was unsuccessful, necessitating open reduction. Periosteal interposition was found in these cases. No reduction was performed in 39 cases. (This includes stage I–IVa injuries).

Peiro et al. (16) treated one three-fragment and one two-fragment fracture

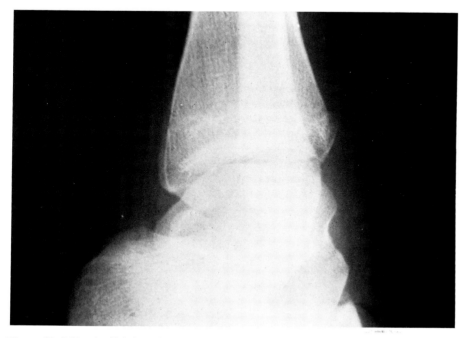

Figure 13–14B A slightly oblique lateral view showing minimal anterior displacement. No other fracture lines are seen on the lateral view as would be the case with a triplane fracture.

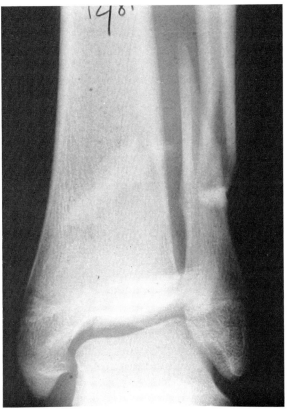 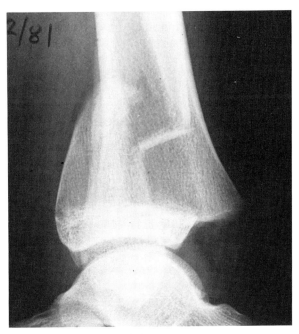

Figure 13–15 A triplane fracture (by operative findings) with an associated fibular fracture. **A** Anteroposterior view.

Figure 13–15B Lateral view.

by closed means, two two-fragment fractures by open methods, and two two-fragment fractures by casting in situ (33% open reductions). Closed treatment consisted of immobilization in a long leg cast, with nonweight-bearing for 4 weeks, followed by a short leg weight-bearing cast for an additional 2–4 weeks. One of the two fragment fractures was fixed with screws alone for the fibula fracture, an anteroposterior screw for the metaphyseal fracture, and a screw for the sagittal fracture at the epiphysis.

Tinnemans and Severijnen's (20) two cases were both treated by closed methods. They believed that with a three-part fracture an associated fibular fracture may prevent closed reduction by maintaining its angular deformity and an open reduction may then be indicated.

Because these fractures generally occur in children with a maturing physis, growth arrest is not a problem but joint incongruity is. Fractures which show 2 mm of more displacement on plain x-rays should have a closed reduction. An adequate closed reduction is defined as that which occurs with satisfactory anesthesia, internal rotation of the foot, and advancement of the fibular-metaphyseal piece anteriorly and the anterior tibial piece posteriorly. If this fails to reduce the fracture or the reduction cannot be maintained in a long leg cast, and there is 2 mm or more of joint incongruity present on either the lateral or anteroposterior roentgenograms, internal fixation should be accomplished. Previously taken tomograms (AP and lateral) and, if possible, a CT scan should be available prior to open reduction so that preoperative planning

Distal Tibial Epiphysis Fractures

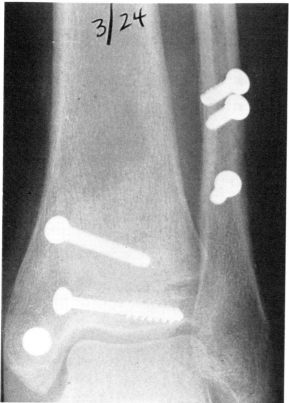

Figure 13–15C At 4 months postoperatively, this anteroposterior view shows the screw fixation for the fibula, posterior metaphyseal piece, epiphysis, and medial malleolus.

Figure 13–15 Lateral view of Figure 15C. (Case courtesy of David Gershuni, M.D., San Diego, California.)

can be done. Depending on the fracture configuration, two incisions may have to be used (anteromedial and anterolateral), and internal fixation both above and below the physis may be necessary, particularly in the three- or four-part triplane fractures.

Associated fibular fractures may have to be internally fixed; if so, provisional fixation may be done first. If the reduction of the tibial fractures is made more difficult by fibular fixation (i.e., periosteal interposition, etc.), the provisional fibular fixation can be released and the tibial fragments internally fixed as a first step. Dias and Giegerich (3) did not find fibular fixation necessary in their two cases. With reference to the tibial fractures, Peiro et al. (16) believed that in the two two-fragment triplanes they operated on "reduction of the anterolateral fragment was unsuccessful . . . when internal fixation of the posterior metaphyseal fragment preceded." Figure 13–15 shows closure of the coronal and sagittal epiphyseal fractures by separate screws to obviate this problem. Fixation of the tibial components can proceed from distal to proximal (intraarticular epiphyseal to metaphyseal) or vice versa depending on the individual fracture. In two-fragment fractures, again depending on the circumstances, metaphyseal fixation alone may produce an anatomic reduction.

Our preference is to use 3.5-mm interfragmentary AO/ASIF cortical screws for the fibula and epiphyseal fractures because they can be easily removed 6–12 weeks postinjury. If a 4.0-mm cancellous screw is used in the epiphysis, it should be removed at 6–8 weeks postinjury. Depending on the size of the metaphyseal fragment, AO/ASIF cancellous screws of 4.0 or 6.5 mm diameter or interfragmentary cortical screws of 3.5 or 4.5 mm can be used—usually inserted in an anteroposterior direction. Smooth pins are less desirable for maintenance of an anatomic reduction because they do not compress the fracture fragments adequately. Intraoperative x-rays are mandatory to determine the adequacy of reduction and the direction and length of the fixation devices. Regardless of postoperative immobilization, weight-bearing other than toe-touching should be delayed for 6 weeks.

Prognosis

Growth arrest is not a problem in most triplane cases, as Karrholm et al. (8) and others have pointed out, and follow-up for that complication is usually not indicated because of the low remaining growth in the tibial physis. In the University of Chicago series (1), three patients had external rotation deformities at follow-up and one had a joint incongruity. All of these complications were related to incomplete reduction of the fracture. Other complications reported by Dias and Giegerich (3) include aching pain after athletic activities in two surgically treated cases and a loss of 5° of ankle motion in another patient. Two of Peiro et al.'s (16) cases had joint incongruity of 1.5 and 1 mm, respectively, although the patients were asymptomatic. As with other intraarticular ankle fractures, a nonanatomic reduction, whether obtained by open or closed methods, is more likely to be symptomatic. The prognosis of triplane fractures then is related directly to the anatomicity and maintenance of the obtained reduction and, in that respect, parallels adult ankle fractures.

Summary

1. Triplane fractures can occur as two-, three-, or four-part fractures with or without a fibular fracture.

2. Diagnosis of the particular anatomy of each fracture is ascertained by plain x-rays; and if the fracture is displaced 2 mm or greater on any x-ray view, AP and lateral tomograms and, if possible, a limited CT scan should be done.

3. Casting in situ for nondisplaced fractures or closed reduction for displaced fractures should be attempted first by internal rotation and anterior movement of the fibular metaphyseal piece. Failure to obtain and/or maintain an adequate closed reduction (less than 2 mm displacement) on plain x-rays is a rationale for operative treatment.

4. Operative treatment consists of screw fixation for the metaphyseal fragment alone, usually in two-part fractures and both metaphyseal and epiphyseal screw fixation in three-part fractures. Associated fibular fractures may also have to be internally fixed.

5. The prognosis is generally good if adequate reduction by closed or open means has been achieved.

REFERENCES

1. Cooperman DR, Spiegel PG, Laros GS (1978). Tibial fractures involving the ankle in children. J Bone Joint Surg 60A:81040–1046.
2. Denton JR, Fischer SJ (1981). The medial triplane fracture: report of an unusual injury. J Trauma 21:991–995.

3. Dias LS, Giegerich CR (1983). Fractures of the distal tibial epiphysis in adolescence. J Bone Joint Surg 65A:438–444.
4. Dias LS, Tachdjian MO (1978). Physeal injuries of the ankle in children. Clin Orthop 136:230–233.
5. Dingeman, RD, Shaver, GB (1978). Operative treatment of displaced Salter-Harris III distal tibial fractures. Clin Orthop 135:101–103.
6. Karrholm J, Hansson LI, Laurin S (1981). Computed tomography of intraarticular supination—eversion fractures of the ankle in adolescents. J Pediatr Orthop 1:181–187.
7. Karrholm J, Hansson LI, Laurin S (1982). Supination-eversion injuries of the ankle in children: a retrospective study of radiographic classification and treatment. J Pediatr Orthop 2:147–159.
8. Karrholm J, Hansson LI, Selvik G (1982). Roentgen stereophotogrammetric analysis of growth pattern after supination—eversion ankle injuries in children. J Pediatr Orthop 2:25–37.
9. Kleiger B, Mankin HJ (1964). Fracture of the lateral portion of the distal tibial epiphysis. J Bone Joint Surg 46A:25–32.
10. Letts RM (1982). The hidden adolescent ankle fracture. J Pediatr Orthop 2:161–164.
11. Lynn MD (1972). The triplane distal tibial epiphyseal fracture. Clin Orthop 86:187–190.
12. MacNealy GA, Rogers LF, Hernandez R et al. (1982). Injuries of the distal tibial epiphysis: systematic radiographic evaluation. Am J Radiol 138:683–689.
13. Marmor L (1970). An unusual fracture of the tibial epiphysis. Clin Orthop 73:132–135.
14. Molster A, Soreide O, Solhaub JH et al. (1977). Fractures of the lateral part of the distal tibial epiphysis (Tillaux or Kleiger fracture). Injury 8:260–263.
15. Ogden JA (1982). Skeletal Injury in the Child. Lea & Febiger, Philadelphia, pp. 596–620.
16. Peiro A, Aracil J, Marto SF et al. (1981). Triplane distal tibial epiphyseal fracture. Clin Orthop 160:196–200.
17. Protas JM, Kornblatt BA (1981). Fractures of the lateral margin of the distal tibia. Diagn Radiol 138:55–57.
18. Rang M (1971). Children's Fractures. Lippincott, Philadelphia, pp. 198–209.
19. Spiegel PG, Cooperman DR, Laros GS (1978). Epiphyseal fractures of the distal ends of the tibia and fibula. J Bone Joint Surg 60A:8:1046–1050.
20. Tinnemans JG, Severijnen RS (1981). The triplane fracture of the distal tibial epiphysis in children. Injury 12:393–396.
21. Torg JS, Ruggiero RA (1975). Comminuted epiphyseal fracture of the distal tibia. Clin Orthop 110:215–217.

Open Reduction and Internal Fixation of Calcaneus Fractures

14

Emile Letournel

The calcaneus has a very complex anatomy, and its articular fractures involve several joints. The surgical approaches are not easy because of skin problems, and its architecture often appears inconvenient for internal fixation. It is probably for these reasons that many physicians treat calcaneus fractures nonoperatively.

It is true that some unreduced calcaneus fractures have an acceptable functional result. The problem is to know how many of the unreduced fractures will achieve no pain, a well-positioned foot, and at least 50% mobility of the subtalar joint. The percentage of those results is less than we can achieve by open reduction and internal fixation.

Open reduction and internal fixation of calcaneus fractures is not a new procedure. Let us remember, however, there are different techniques to reduce the posterior subtalar articular surface and to maintain it reduced using an internal fixation device with bone grafts.

The posterior subtalar articular surface was called the "thalamus" by Destot, and in this chapter we speak of pre-, trans-, or retrothalamic fracture lines.

In 1921 Leriche (4) used a horizontal screw beneath the sustentaculum tali or maintained the reduction of the articular surface with a staple. In 1928 Lenormant and Wilmoth (3) used osteoperiosteal grafts from the external malleolus to sustain the thalamus reduction. In 1948 Palmer (5) modified Lenormant and Wilmoth's technique by using a carved iliac graft to maintain the thalamus. In 1953 Judet et al. (2) suggested that the subtalar joint be reduced anatomically and the reduction maintained by either direct screw fixation or by using the compression effect of a transverse screw passing through a piece of banked cortical bone under the sustentaculum. Later they changed this technique by not using the bank bone graft but instead used isolated screws or screwed plates.

Our personal philosophy follows these principles, but we also emphasize that the isolated reconstruction of the subtalar joint is not enough and that we must reconstruct the whole morphology of the bone in order to restore

173

not only the anatomy of the three articular surfaces of the calcaneus but also their respective orientations. By doing this the congruence of both the subtalar and calcaneus cuboid joints is restored, which in turn allows complete functional mobility.

As always when complex bones are fractured, the first difficulty arises if there is not perfect understanding of the fracture on the preoperative x-rays. A perfect reconstruction is not possible if we do not have in mind an exact representation of the fracture on which we will operate. The preoperative analysis of a calcaneus fracture needs at least two good x-rays: (a) the exact lateral profile of the foot; and (b) the dorsoplantar retrotibial view. The latter view must show the entire fractured calcaneus as well as all parts of the subtalar joint. For this view, the x-ray beam is less oblique than for the Harris-Beath view. These views will suffice with experience, but further help in understanding the fractures is afforded by frontal, profile, or horizontal tomographic views (*1*). A careful analysis of these x-rays with the aid of tracing paper allows the surgeon to classify exactly the fracture to be treated.

Classification

All displaced calcaneus fractures have in common one fracture line, the *separation fracture* (Figure 14–1). This fracture line is oblique frontward and outward on the upper aspect of the bone and upward and outward on the retrotibial aspect. It breaks the upper aspect of the bone either through the sinus tarsi, always behind the interosseous ligament, or through the subtalar articular surface (i.e., the thalamus). This is appreciated on the retrotibial view, which also clearly

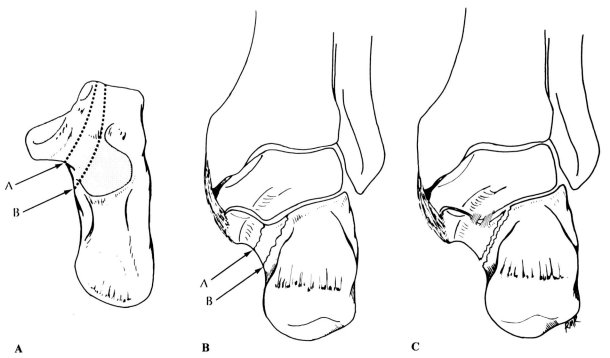

Figure 14–1 The constant separation fracture line. **A** The fracture runs through the sinus tarsi behind the interosseous ligament. **B** The fracture intersects the thalamus. **C** A two fragment fracture without displacement (exceptional).

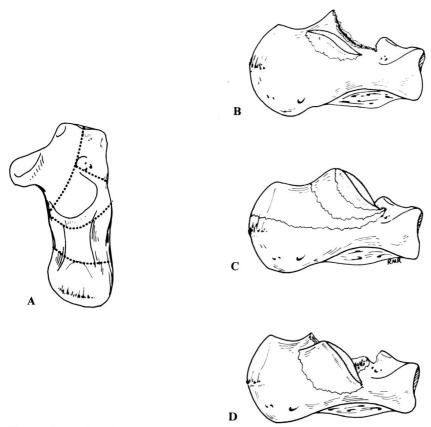

Figure 14–2 Three-fragment fractures. **A** Impaction of the thalamus: the various fracture lines (seen from above). **B** Horizontal impaction of the thalamus. **C** Possible fracture lines of a vertical impaction. **D** Vertical impaction of the thalamus.

shows the rupture of the internal aspect of the calcaneus (Figure 14–1b). An essential point is that this fragment remains perfectly connected to the talus by the interosseous ligaments (Figure 14–1c) and thus is the key for the reconstruction. This constant fracture line divides the calcaneus into two parts. It is highly unusual for the trauma to end here because most of the time there are additional fractures.

In the simplest cases, the trauma adds an impaction of the posterior subtalar articular surface (i.e., thalamus) (Figure 14–2A), but the general morphology of the bone itself is preserved; particularly, the inferior cortex is not ruptured. These are the three-fragment fractures. The subtalar impaction or thalamic impaction is best appreciated on the lateral profile and may be either: (a) horizontal, the articular surface being freed between the separation fracture and a retrothalamic fracture (Figure 14–2B); or (b) vertical (Figure 14–2C,D); here the posterior fracture line freeing the articular surface may be immediately posterior to it, may divide the upper aspect of the tuberosity, or less commonly is horizontally disposed, starting from the sinus tarsi and finishing at the posterior aspect of the bone, just above the Achilles tendon insertion. These are the "tongue-type" fractures (Figures 14–3, 14–4). A vertical impaction limited posteriorly by a fracture line cutting the upper aspect of the tuberosity is shown in Figure 14–5.

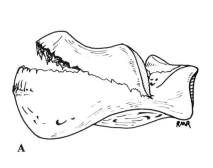
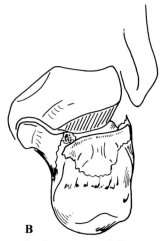

Figure 14–3 A type of vertical impaction of the thalamus: the "tongue type" fracture. **A** A profile view. **B** The tongue seen from behind.

The complex cases (Figure 14–6) comprise four fragments or more, including the inner and undisplaced fragment separated by the basic fracture line and the impacted thalamus. Other fragments are delineated by additional frontal or sagittal fracture lines which divide the inferior cortex of the bone. These fractures compromise the whole morphology of the bone and especially the relative relationship between the three poles of the bone: the center of the subtalar joint, the apophysis, and the tuberosity (Figure 14–7). Whether it is included in simple or complex fractures, the thalamic impaction always has the same features. This thalamic impaction into the underlying cancellous bone produces enlargment of the bone, and the external cortex may literally explode. Usually (Figure 14-8) it breaks into several parts, but there is always an important fragment comprising the upper part of this face and a few millimeters of the subtalar articular surface along its upper border (Figure 14–6A,B). However, in "tongue-type" fractures (Figure 14–9), the impacted thalamus brings with it the upper part of the external cortex (Figure 14-10).

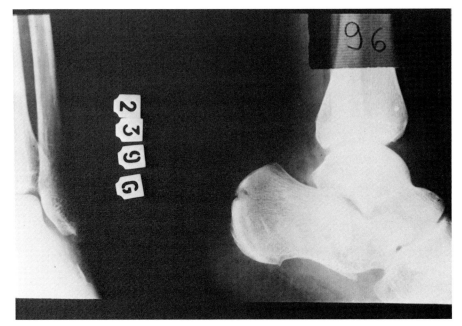

Figure 14–4 Profile view of a typical "tongue type" fracture.

Calcaneus Fractures

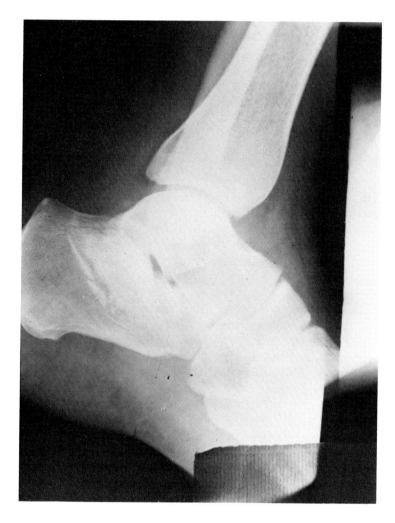

Figure 14–5 Vertical impaction of the thalamus limited posteriorly by a fracture line cutting the upper aspect of the tuberosity.

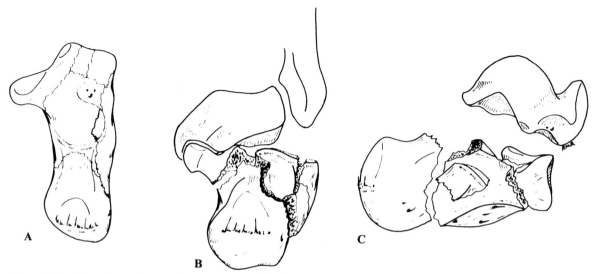

Figure 14–6 Complex calcaneus fractures comprising four fragments or more. **A** Fracture lines on the upper aspect of the bone. **B** The fracture seen from behind. **C** Profile of the same case.

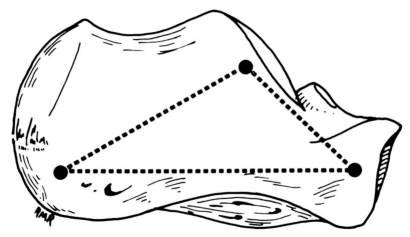

Figure 14-7 The three poles of the calcaneus.

Today we see more complex cases in which it is always easy to identify the subtalar impaction, but there are many other fracture lines which divide the remaining part of the calcaneus in many fragments or pieces, sometimes innumerable, and the fracture cannot be classified other than as comminuted (Figure 14-11).

Unusually, as reported by Warrich and Bremer (6), we observe a displaced fracture with just two fragments (Figure 14-12). After the separation fracture, the posteroexternal fragment bearing the subtalar articular surface, thanks to

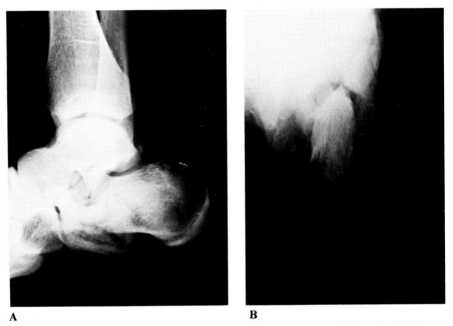

Figure 14-8A Complex fracture with a vertical impaction of the thalamus limited posteriorly by a fracture line cutting the upper aspect of the tuberosity. **B** Retrotibial view shows clearly the disjunction of the subtalar joint and enlargement of the bone.

Calcaneus Fractures

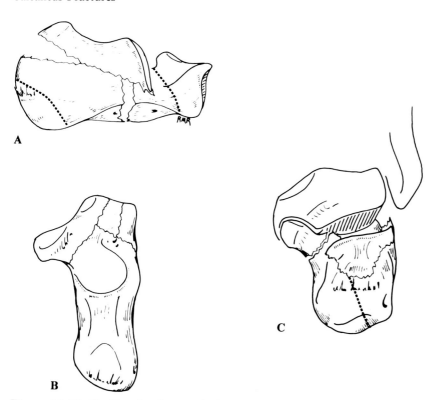

Figures 14–9A–C Complex fracture including a "tongue-type" impaction of the thalamus. **C** Note that the thalamus impaction brings with it the upper part of the external cortex of the bone.

the rupture of the subtalar ligaments, displaces outwardly and in supination does not sustain any more fractures, and dislocates laterally.

Surgical Treatment

All the displaced articular fractures are operated on with a strong internal fixation in order to restore the normal anatomy and allow immediate mobilization of the joint with the avoidance of stiffening plasters. Early operations, performed as soon as possible after the accident, are probably ideal; however, these are difficult operations and are not to be performed as an emergency measure by insufficiently experienced surgeons.

If edema or fracture blisters are present, the operation must be postponed and the leg placed in an elevated position. It is prudent to wait 4–6 days or more until the edema subsides and the skin becomes normal again before operating.

The Operation

The patient lies on the uninjured side on an ordinary table. The foot rests on its inner face on a dense cushion; a tourniquet is used routinely. The surgical approach is critical because one of the major problems postoperatively is skin

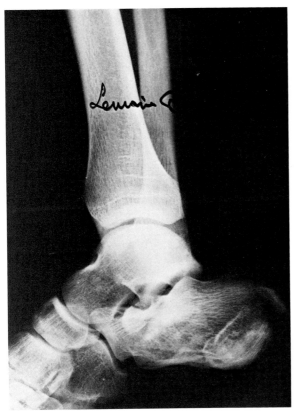

Figure 14–10A X-ray view of a complex fracture including a "tongue-type" impaction.

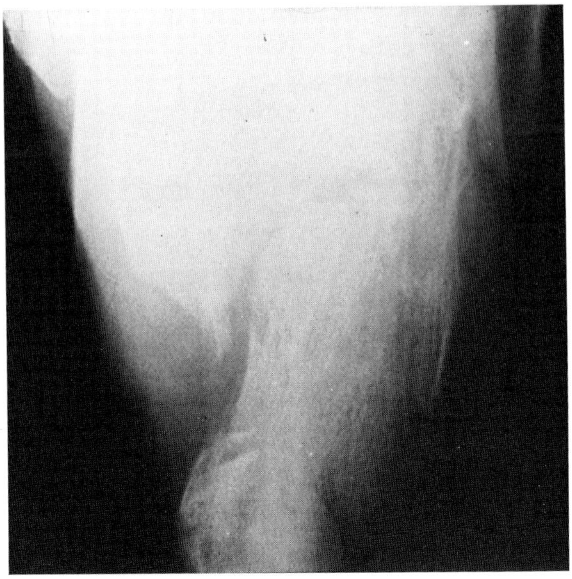

Figure 14–10B Another view of the same fracture.

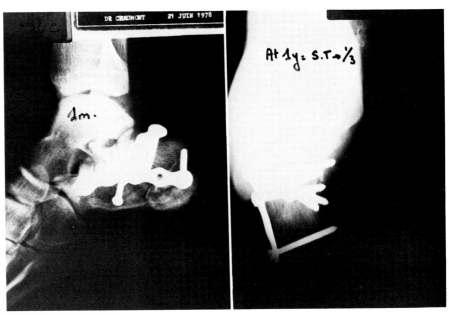

Figure 14–10C Appearance of the same fracture at 1 year after surgery. The subtalar joint mobility is one-third normal.

Calcaneus Fractures

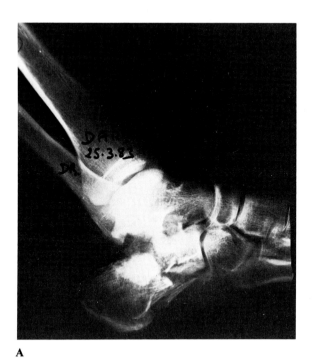

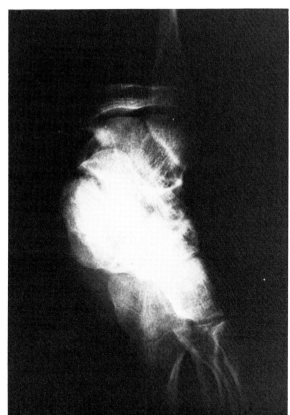

Figure 14–11 A very complex (i.e., comminuted) fracture of the calcaneus. **A** Profile view. **B** Retrotibial view. **C** Tomography.

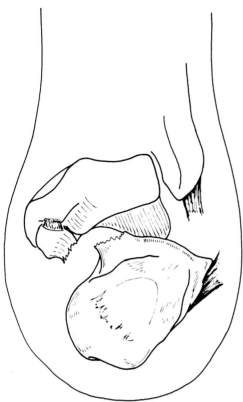

Figure 14–12A Two-fragment fracture of the calcaneus. The inner fragment remains connected to the talus. The external one is dislocated outwardly.

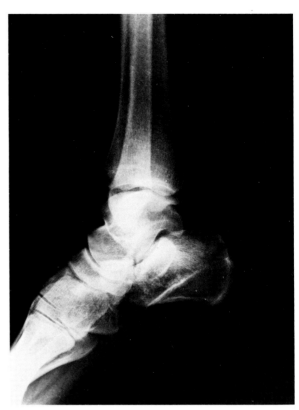

Figure 14–12B Profile x-ray view of a two-fragment fracture.

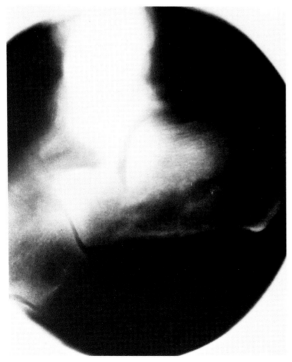

Figure 14–12C Profile tomography of a two-fragment fracture.

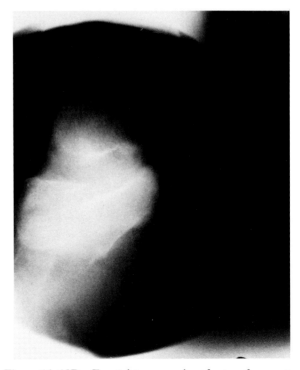

Figure 14–12D Frontal tomography of a two-fragment fracture.

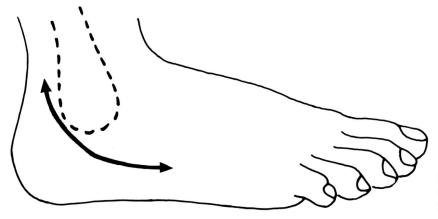

Figure 14–13 The incision we routinely use to fix calcaneus fractures.

necrosis. For that reason, we routinely use a retro- and sublateral malleolar incision along the distal border of the peroneal tendons (Figure 14–13). Once the skin is incised, the sural nerve is avoided, and the knife tries to reach the calcaneal cortex by the shortest route in order to avoid damage from retractors applied to the skin edges. Then all the soft parts, especially the peroneal tendons with their sheaths, are elevated from the outer aspect of the bone. The peroneal calcaneus ligament is cut, which opens the subtalar joint. If the displaced thalamus takes a part of the external cortex with it, as in Figure 14–9, the impaction is immediately obvious. However, if the impaction does not comprise the external border of the thalamus, as shown on Figure 14–6, we incline the upper fragment of the outer cortex outward and downward to see the subtalar joint impaction.

Reduction and fixation must have two objectives: to restore the congruency of the subtalar and calcaneocuboid joints, and to reestablish the general morphology of the calcaneus by restoring the position of the subtalar joint surface relative to the apophysis and the tuberosity (Figure 14–7).

The first action consists of restoring the posterior subtalar joint (Figure 14–14) with a spatula or a curved chisel introduced under the impacted fragment (Figure 14–14A). The impaction is progressively reduced and the articular frag-

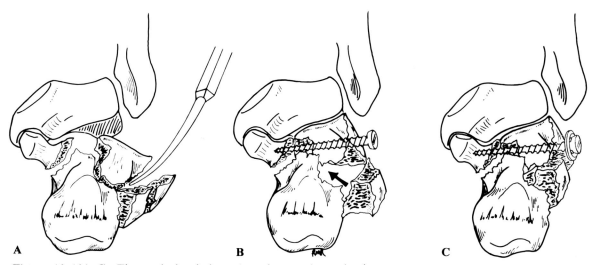

Figures 14–14A–C The surgical technique. A washer may be used to increase transverse compression effect.

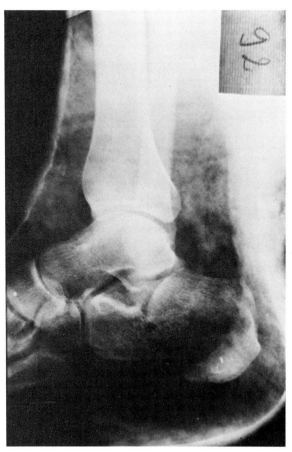

Figure 14–15A Two-fragment fracture with vertical impaction of the thalamus.

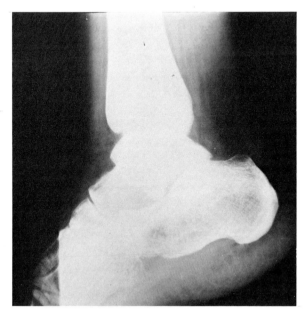

Figure 14–15B The result at 5 years after fixation by an isolated screw.

ment brought back against the talus. We then check that the disimpacted block is level with the part of the thalamus belonging to the internal undisplaced separated fragment. If an external cortical fragment brings a few millimeters of articular surface with it, it is then reduced to complete the reconstruction of the subtalar joint. Fixation is achieved by means of isolated screws (3.6 or 4 mm), which go through the reduced fragments and take a firm hold into the inner cortex of the separated fragment (Figure 14–14B). If the quality of the external cortex fragment is not excellent or if we want to increase the transverse compression effect, screws may be inserted with a washer (Figure 14–14C). This screw fixation of the impacted subtalar joint fragment may suffice in two- or three-fragment fractures, allowing us to have as little foreign material as possible, a distinct advantage in this area with very susceptible skin. Figure 14–15 shows such an example and the result at 5 years.

In complex fractures with additional frontal or sagittal fracture lines which delineate many fragments, the reconstruction and fixation of the subtalar joint with screws, as described above, is always the first stage of the operation. This is followed by reconstruction of the other parts of the calcaneus. Further reduction is gained by putting the foot in equinus and afterward in valgus while retracting the tuberosity backward. This maneuver may be facilitated by introducing a big Lambotte's hook along the upper face of the calcaneus in front of the Achilles' tendon or, exceptionally, by exerting traction on a temporary insertion of a Kirschner wire transfixing the tuberosity.

Calcaneus Fractures

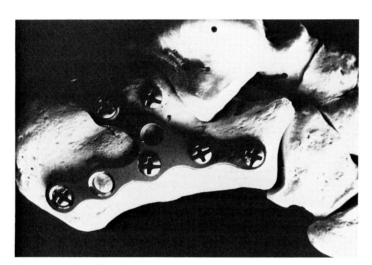
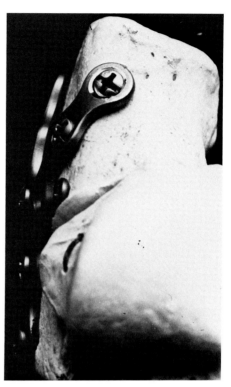

Figure 14–16 The Y-plate applied on a dry bone. **A** Lateral view.

Figure 14–16B Seen from above, the upper branch of a Y-plate rests on the upper aspect of the tuberosity.

It is essential to restore the normal angulation between the subtalar joint and the apophysis because a perfectly restored subtalar joint embedded into the calcaneus does not yield a good result.

The reduction is fixed by a plate, and for these complex cases we have been using, for years, a "Y" vitallium plate (Figure 14–16). The upper branch is bent so as to be parallel to the subtalar joint and to have its last screw hole on the upper aspect of the bone. The screws through the holes of this branch reinforce the subtalar joint fixation. The inferior branch of the plate is applied on the tuberosity passing under the peroneal tendons. Two or three screws, inserted into the tuberosity, usually give good fixation. It is not always possible to insert the distal screw without risk to the skin, or it may be done through a separate puncture of the skin. The distal branch of the Y-plate approximately follows the axis of the great apophysis; two screws are usually sufficient. Figure 14–17 shows such an example and the results at 3.5 years. In some cases with multiple splits into the great apophysis, as in the case shown in Figure 14–18, the plate may span the calcaneocuboid joint space and one screw is inserted into the cuboid. The plate must be removed after healing. The most complex cases require more complex internal fixation. Besides using the Y-plate, some lag screws of different diameters are needed to fix secondary fracture lines, as shown in Figures 14–19 and 14–20.

It is important to state that we do not use any cancellous bone grafts to fill the gap created by the reduction of the impacted fragment. Once the reduction is achieved, the repositioning of the fragment of the outer cortex of the bone partially fills the loss of substance; in practice, reconstruction of the spongiosa trabeculae occurs quickly, and we have not observed secondary impactions if the internal fixation was done correctly.

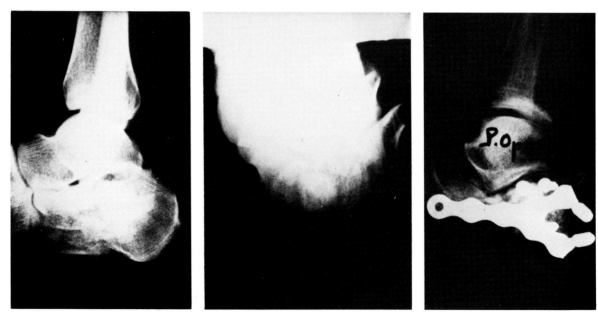

Figure 14–17A A complex fracture fixed with a Y-plate and its postoperative appearance.

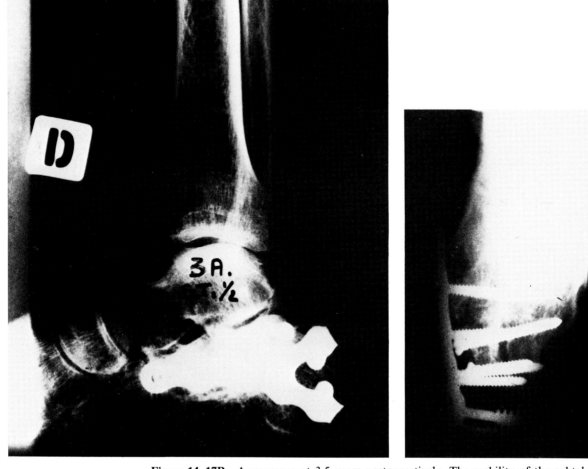

Figure 14–17B Appearance at 3.5 years postoperatively. The mobility of the subtalar joint is one-half normal.

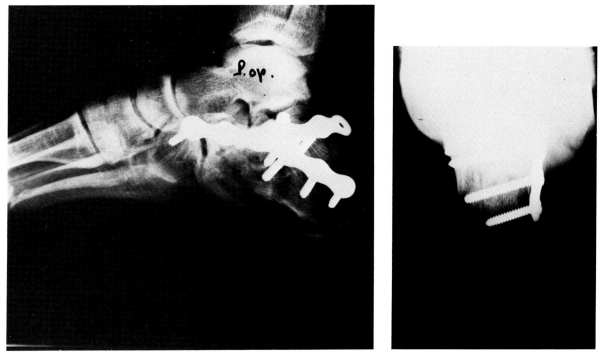

Figures 14–18A,B Postoperative appearance of the case shown in Figure 14–8.

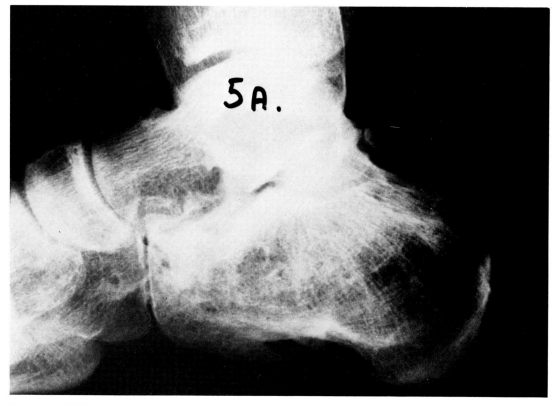

Figure 14–18C Appearance 5 years postoperatively. The plate was removed 1 year after surgery. The subtalar joint is mobile at one-third normal.

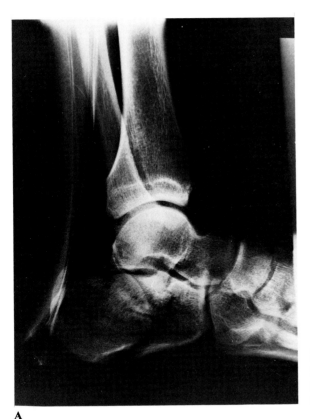

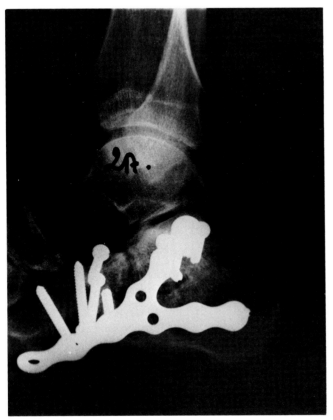

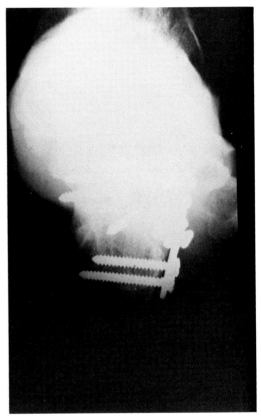

Figure 14–19 A complex fracture with horizontal impaction of the thalamus. **A** Profile view. **B,C** Appearance 2 years postoperatively. The mobility of the subtalar joint is more than two-thirds normal.

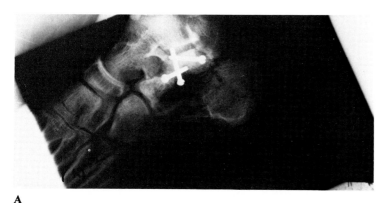
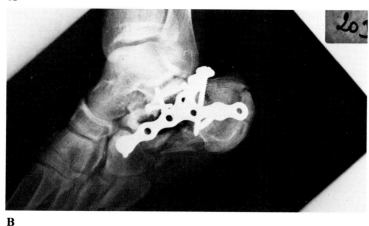

Figure 14–20 Postoperative appearance of the case shown on Figure 14–11. **A** Intraoperative view after reconstruction of the thalamus with isolated screws. In fact, the thalamus was divided into four parts. **B** Appearance 3 weeks postoperatively. This is a recent case, and weight bearing was allowed at the beginning of July 1983.

Closure must be done very carefully with atraumatic needles—without using forceps to hold the skin and without overtightening the stitches. A suction drain is used routinely, and the foot is maintained in an elevated position for about 3 days. Passive mobilization begins on the third day, and active mobilization on about the eighth day. Full weight-bearing is allowed by the 90th day.

Results

The first reference here is to Judet's departmental statistics published when I was his assistant at Raymond Poincare Hospital at the end of the 1970s. There were 83 cases having a follow-up period of more than 2 years in that study. Postoperative complications included skin necrosis, which led in some instances to an infection. Among 83 cases, eight patients had skin necrosis and three a severe infection; these are among the fair or poor results. A wide debridement of the infection followed by closure over several suction drains and a modification of the internal fixation (Figure 14–21) were needed to cure the infection, but the subtalar joint always remained stiff.

The long term results were as follows:

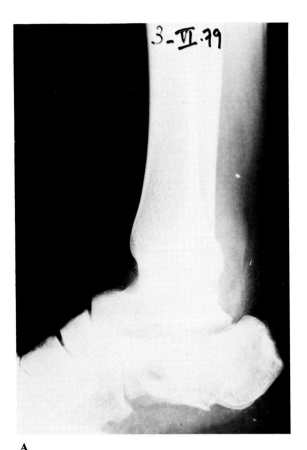
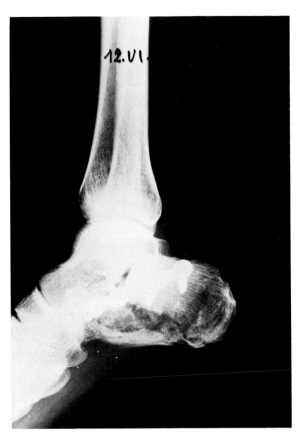

Figures 14–21A,B Very complex fracture of the calcaneus with vertical impaction. Postoperative appearance after the first attempt at internal fixation. The initial operation was followed by an acute infection, after which the case was referred to us. We undertook complete debridement and changed the internal fixation.

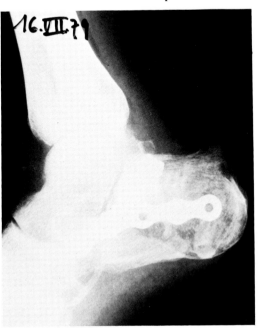
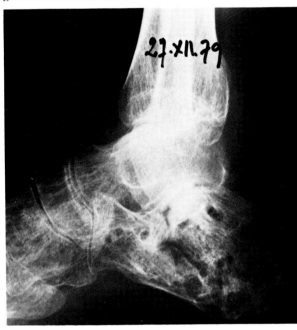

Figures 14–21C,D Postoperative appearance: The plate was removed 5 months after the debridement. In spite of that, the subtalar joint remained stiff.

Calcaneus Fractures

Very good—23 (26%): no pain, normal walking and running, easy walking on tiptoe

Good—24 (30%): occasional pain, running and walking without limit, can stand all day

Fair—27 (33%): pain while walking on uneven ground, cannot run easily, cannot walk on tiptoe

Bad—9 (10%): comprising three infections, six technical failures

On the whole, 56% of the patients had either no functional disability or, at the maximum, occasional pain while walking on uneven ground.

The comparison between anatomic and functional results proved that:

Very good results—23: very good reductions

Good results—24: 22 very good reductions and two slightly—imperfect ones

Fair results—27: no one had a very good reduction

Bad results—9: there were seven technical failures

The condition of the subtalar joint was noted in the 83 cases of Judet's department and the 16 cases operated on at Choisy, all of which needed a Y-plate fixation. We found that of the 99 cases:

3 Cases had a normal joint

14 Had a mobility of three-fourths normal

30 Had a mobility of one-half normal

36 Had a mobility of one-fourth normal

16 Had a stiff subtalar joint

On the whole, 47 cases (47%) had a useful mobility of the subtalar joint.

Conclusions

The surgical treatment has two goals: (a) to restore the normal anatomy of the calcaneus and the foot; and (b) to maintain the subtalar joint mobility. Concerning the first point, seven of the 99 cases noted above were considered technical failures, with some undergoing an arthrodesis of the posterior subtalar joint. A very good reduction of both the calcaneus and the subtalar joint was obtained in 55% of the cases, and 56% of the patients obtained a very good functional result.

With regard to subtalar joint mobility, at the beginning of this series some internal fixations were not completely reliable, and a plaster cast was applied with its subsequent consequences for subtalar joint mobility. Currently, since better reductions are being achieved and rigidly fixed with immediate mobilization, the recovery of the subtalar joint mobility is anticipated more regularly. Nevertheless, only three cases out of the 99 have a normal joint, and 47% have a mobility of half normal or more, 36% have very restricted mobility, and 16% have a stiff joint.

Are these results worthwhile, and is this difficult surgery advisable? I think that these restricted mobilities, in spite of the early mobilization, are due to small errors in the orientation of the reconstructed subtalar joint relative to other articular surfaces of the bone. More care, better internal fixation, improved devices, and routine intraoperative x-ray control are necessary to improve the results.

A normal life and sports participation are possible with a subtalar joint mobile at half of its normal range of motion. A joint mobility of even one-

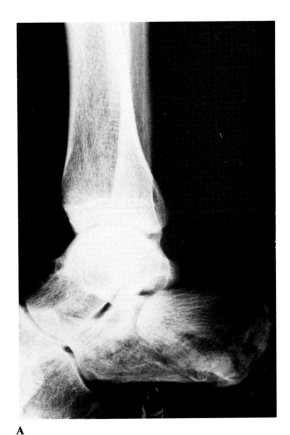 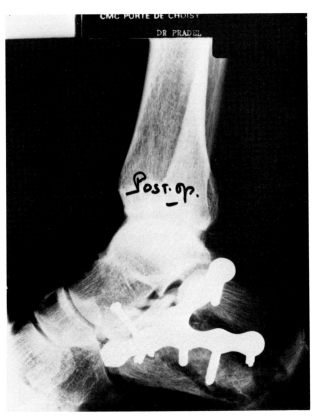

Figure 14–22A Complex fracture with vertical impaction. **B** Postoperative appearance demonstrating that we performed an overreduction and that the calcaneus has not recovered its normal anatomy.

third or one-fourth normal also appears useful and is valuable in terms of allowing the patient to walk on uneven ground much better than ankylosis of the subtalar joint would allow.

Fifty-six percent of good or very good functional results and 47% of subtalar joints recovering more than half of their mobility may appear as already better than the results of nonoperative methods. Nevertheless, these results need to be improved and I am sure that the solution lies in perfect reduction of the bone, which is sometimes difficult to achieve. The reduction shown in Figure 14–22 would now not be acceptable because the normal relationship between the three poles of the bone was not restored.

REFERENCES

1. Champetier J, et al. (1979). Fracture articulaire du calcaneum-interet des tomographies horizontales pour le diagnostic. Presse Med 7–8:753.
2. Judet R, Judet J, Lagrange J (1954). Traitement des fractures du calcaneum comportant une disjonction astraga-lo-calcaneum. Mem Acad Chir 80:158–160.
3. Lenormant W, et al. (1928) Concerning the surgical treatment of fractures of the calcis. Bulletin et memoires de la Sociéte Nationale de Chirurgie 54:1353–1355.
4. Leriche R (1922) Osteosynthese pour fracture par ecrasement du calcaneum à sept fragments, Lyon Chir 559.
5. Palmer I (1948). The mechanism and treatment of fractures of calcaneus—open reduction with the use of cancellous grafts. J Bone Joint Surg 30A:2–8.
6. Warrick CK, Brenner AE (1953). Fractures of the calcaneus. J Bone Joint Surg 35B:33–49.

Internal Fixation of Nonunions After Unsuccessful Electromagnetic Stimulation

15

Howard Rosen

The use of electricity to treat fractures that fail to unite goes back at least to the beginning of the nineteenth century (*14,15,19*). At that time galvanic current was used through transcutaneous electrodes inserted into the fracture areas while the limb was immobilized with splints. Clinical success was reported with such treatment, although x-rays were not available then for confirmation.

Electricity and its effect on fracture healing and bone formation was rediscovered about 30 years ago (*11,26*) and specifically began to be used for clinical nonunion problems about 10 years ago (*5,8*). Three major clinical methods have evolved and are in use today.

Methods of Electrical Stimulation

The invasive method of Paterson et al. (*18*) requires an operative procedure with the implantation of a coiled cathode wire into the nonunion area and an implantable anode and battery in adjacent muscle connected by insulated leads to the cathode. The battery is removed after 4 months when the fracture should be united. Casts are used for immobilization until fracture healing occurs.

With the semi-invasive system of Brighton et al. (*7*), usually four insulated cathode electrode wires are inserted percutaneously under fluoroscopic control across the nonunion site and are connected to an external battery power source and generator. This allows 20 μA of direct current to be transmitted across the nonunion. The limb is immobilized in a plaster cast, a brace, or with external fixators. Modifications of this system to electrify Steinman pins (*12*) (part of an external fixator system), plates and screws, or intramedullary rods (*13*) have also been developed to bring electrical current to the nonunion site. The overall success rate with this varied group of electrical stimulation techniques for the treatment of nonunions is about 85%.

Finally, a totally non-invasive system using pulsing electromagnetic fields (PEMF) to induce an electrical current across the nonunion area and thus influence its union was conceived by Bassett about 13 years ago (3). Experimental proof of the biological activity of this PEMF system in tissue cultures and animal experiments preceded the use of this method in clinical nonunions. A number of clinical trials during the past 5 years have shown evidence of about an 80–85% success rate (6) with this method if a specific protocol is adhered to: (a) application of a snug plaster cast to control motion; (b) careful measurements of cast diameter to establish intercoil distances so that the units could be set for the proper pulse generation; (c) placement of parallel coils across the fracture by x-ray control; (d) treatment at home with the unit plugged into an electrical outlet for 10–12 hr/day; (e) no weight-bearing until some union is attained by (f) serial x-rays; and finally (g) protected gradual rehabilitative weight-bearing as early union occurs.

Healing of Nonunions: Theoretical Concepts

How does PEMF work? Bassett et al. (2) postulated that selective control of mesenchymal cells can be achieved by programming pulsed electrical events in the cells' inner environment. With nonunions the signal used induces fibrocartilage to calcify in the gap between the nonunited bone fragments. The cartilage and soft tissue which impede vascular invasion and osteogenesis in nonunions become calcified under PEMF treatment. Once this occurs, vascular invasion, chondroclasis, and replacement by bone follows, healing the fracture. This process is similar to normal endochondral ossification that spontaneously occurs in stages in fresh fracture healing.

It is also of interest to note that in the experiments of Müller et al. (16) and Schenk (23) hypertrophic nonunions were created in the radius of dogs by constant mechanical instability, resulting in the development of fibrocartilage and fibrous tissue between the bone ends. These investigators then applied a compression plate to stabilize these experimental hypertrophic nonunions. The unmineralized cartilage and fibrous tissue in the interfragmentary gap began to mineralize as a result of the stability gained by the plate. This was caused by chondrocyte-mediated mineralization, which appeared as early as 6 weeks after the rigid fixation plate was applied. No resection of the pseudarthrosis tissue, no bone graft, and no cast were necessary to achieve union in these experiments. The mineralized fibrocartilage then formed columns which by vascular ingrowth of osteoblasts, formed woven bony trabeculae (third to eighth week). This woven bone was then remodeled into mature lamellar cancellous bone by the eighth to 16th week; and it was reconstructed into cortical compact bone by 16–24 weeks.

This brief review gives some insight into the present theory of the healing of nonunions induced by electricity with cast immobilization or immobilization by stable internal fixation with a plate. Both apparently induce calcification of the avascular fibrocartilage.

Results of PEMF and Operative Treatment of Nonunions

The results of a large multicenter series of PEMF-treated nonunions were reported by Bassett et al. in 1982 (6). There were 1,007 nonunited fractures and 71 failed arthrodeses with an average healing rate of 81% at Columbia Presbyterian Medical Center, 79% internationally, and 76% in the rest of the United States. There was a 75% success rate in a subset of 332 nonunions with an average of 4.7 years' disability, an average of 3.4 previous operative failures, and a 35% rate of infection. Total knee prosthesis failures with failed arthrodesis were fused with PEMF in 85% of patients.

Let us compare these statistics with some series of operative treatment of nonunions and pseudarthroses. Weber and Brunner (24) reported that 126 of 127 noninfected nonunions of the tibia achieved union (99.2%) by operative stable internal fixation. Of 122 infected nonunions of the tibia, 117 resulted in sound union (95.9%). In another series by the same authors from 1972 to 1980, 111 noninfected and 35 infected nonunions achieved union with the same success rate (24). Rosen (21,22) reported on the treatment of 122 pseudarthroses and delayed unions of which 24 were infected; 92.6% healed primarily with one internal fixation operation. Most did not require excision of the pseudarthrosis, bone grafts, or casts.

As early as 1965 Anderson et al. (1) reported union in 88.5% of 69 nonunions treated with compression plates, and that same year Müller (17) reported 100 nonunions treated with internal fixation with 97% success. Bone grafts were used as necessary in all of these operative series, especially in atrophic or infected cases. Compression plates, intramedullary rods, or occasionally external fixators were used for fixation. Shingling of infected and atrophic nonunions was also employed.

As one can readily see, nonunion can be treated electrically with about 80% overall success and by modern internal fixation methods with a success rate well within the 90–95% range. What are the fundamental differences between these two methods aside from the above success rates?

Problems With Electricity

Electricity usually does not work with gaps of more than 1 cm in width, in synovial pseudarthrosis, and where motion at the fracture is difficult to control with casts or braces, i.e., in the proximal femur or humerus. Infected draining nonunions seem to do well with PEMF but do not heal well with transcutaneous electrodes. Atrophic and hypertrophic lesions were not differentiated in the above series (3,6) of electrically treated nonunions, nor were the difficult group of metaphyseal-epiphyseal nonunions tabulated or differentiated. We believe that the atrophic and metaphyseal groups represent the more difficult nonunions and should be singled out for special tabulation when reporting on any series of nonunions by electrical or operative means.

Malunion and shortening are not corrected by electricity and are real contraindications for its use. Finally, the long periods of immobilization in plaster casts with non-weight-bearing (which averaged 5.2 to 8.1 months in various series) (3,6) and being plugged into the wall outlet for 10–12 hr a day add immeasurably to the inconvenience of the electrical treatment. This long cast immobilization also gives rise to joint stiffness, osteoporosis, muscle atrophy, and swelling. It is this loss of function as well as joint and limb deformity and disability that should be addressed when comparing the "healing" statistics of the various methods of nonunion treatment. It is not only the healing of the bone but the patient's overall functional result when utilizing the limb that should be considered when evaluating the final results of a therapeutic modality.

Table 15–1 Author's Classification of Acquired Nonunions

I. Degree	III. Callus
A. Delayed union	A. Hypertrophic (vascular—elephant foot)
B. Nonunion	B. Atrophic (hypovascular—nonreactive)
1. Mobile—gap	IV. Infection
2. Immobile	A. Noninfected
C. Pseudarthrosis	B. Infected
1. Synovial	1. Nondraining
II. Site	2. Draining
A. Diaphyseal (shaft)	
1. Nondisplaced	
2. Displaced	
B. Metaphyseal	
1. Intraarticular	

Rationale for Operative Treatment

The rationale for the operative treatment of nonunions is based on cause and classification (Table 15–1). The causes of nonunion are a gap, unbridled motion, loss of blood supply, and possibly infection.

Most fractures of long bones will unite by closed treatment with callus formation in a reasonable time. By 6 months almost all fractures that are going to heal have healed or show progressive healing by serial x-rays. Delayed union means that the fracture is taking longer to unite than would ordinarily be expected for a similar fracture. Nonunion refers to an arrest of the bony fracture repair process (usually 8–9 months after the fracture) and the formation of a fibrous cartilagenous tissue, instead of bone, between the fracture ends. If this nonunion does not heal, motion and shear will cause the formation of a neoarthrosis, a synovial false joint, or pseudarthrosis. Operation or other intervention must supervene to heal this false joint because it will not unite by itself.

Synovial Pseudarthrosis

The diagnosis of a synovial pseudarthrosis is made today by the use of radioisotope studies in addition to standard radiographs (Figure 15.1), stress motion films, and fluoroscopy. According to Esterhai et al. (*10*), in a series of 157 cases one of three patterns were seen using ^{99m}Tc scintigraphy: (a) an intense uniformly increased uptake at the nonunion site (69.5%); (b) a photon-deficient (cold) cleft between intense areas of uptake (23.4%); and (c) indeterminate patterns (7.1%). Those with a cold cleft correlated closely with the presence of synovial pseudarthrosis at surgery.

Diagnostic Tools Used in Nonunions

Other diagnostic tools are used to determine which delayed unions might spontaneously unite. These are osteomedulloangiography (*9*) and intraosseous venography (*20*). Both of these methods have been used to determine the prognosis for healing of fractures and therefore the proper modality of therapy to be used. When angiography was performed at 6 weeks, fractures that would be expected to heal normally already showed reestablishment of the medullary circulation. When fractures showing delayed union were tested at 3 months,

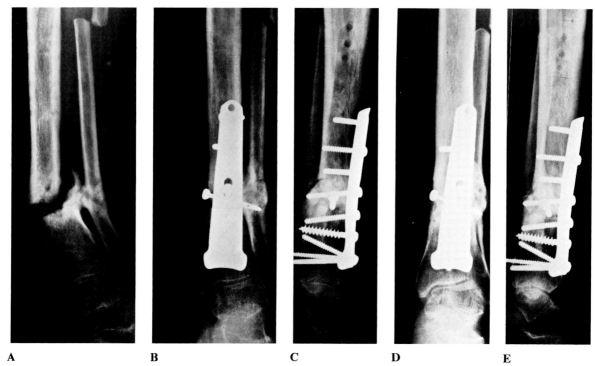

Figure 15–1 This 27-year-old male was struck by a bulldozer in October 1978. He had an open fracture which was treated with pins, a cast, and two plastic operations. In August 1979 he had Hoffman fixation with an iliac bone graft. In July 1980 drainage started. PEMF was applied from July to October 1980. **A** November 1980. He had drainage, motion, 3-cm shortening, a stiff ankle, a valgus external rotation deformity, a gap, oligotrophic pseudarthrosis, and poor dorsiflexion. **B,C** AP and lateral views in April 1981, 2 months postoperatively: osteotomy of the distal fibula, iliac bone graft, AO spoon plate and lag screws, and shingling. No cast was applied. He exercised and used crutches, with 25 lb weight-bearing until he healed. **D,E** Anteroposterior (AP) and lateral views in January 1982, 11 months postoperatively. The fracture healed after 8 months. He now has 75% motion of the ankle and is walking well.

those with reestablished circulation healed well by nonoperative therapy. Those that showed incomplete revascularization required bone grafting to unite them. When venography was used, at 6–8 months those with reconstituted circulation united with electricity and further cast treatment, and those with inadequate revascularization required further surgery and bone grafting. The disadvantages of these methods are that they are invasive, painful procedures that require anesthesia and subjective roentgenographic interpretation rather than quantitative assessment. The results with the above methods are more valuable when they show the circulation to be continuous rather than when they show a failure of revascularization.

Classification of Nonunions

Weber and Cech (25) utilized radioisotope studies in addition to standard radiographs to differentiate the two major categories of their classification: (a) nonunions with vital bone ends, i.e., with good vascularity; (b) nonunions with poor or no blood supply.

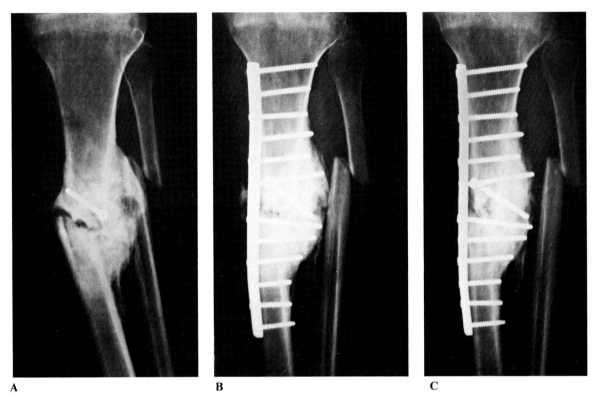

Figure 15–2 This 34-year-old male (260 lb, 6 feet 3 inches in height) was struck by a car in September 1979. He was treated with a compression plate which broke 4 months later. In February 1980 the metal was removed and a bone graft, brace, and cast were applied; he underwent another bone graft in September 1980. PEMF was applied from February to December 1981 with a cast and no weight-bearing. **A** February 1982. At 2.5 years after the fracture. Note the hypertrophic nonunion with a medial gap, valgus deformity, and the old screw. **B** February 1982. Note the postoperative correction of valgus, the AO tension band plate, lag screw fixation, and shingling. No bone graft and no cast were used. **C** March 1983, 13 months postoperatively. He was healed at 9 months, walking without aids, and he had good function.

Those with good blood supply respond by forming callus: a large amount is called an "elephant's foot" (Figure 15–2); a smaller amount is called a "horse's foot"; and poor or no callus but vital ends on the bone scan is called an oligotrophic nonunion (Figure 15–3).

Those fractures with a poor blood supply show failure of callus formation (Figure 15–4). Those with partially or totally nonunited avascular butterfly fragments or segments fall into this group, as do those with a gap caused by a fibrous defect or synovial pseudarthrosis. Infected cases may be in either category, but these usually show a great deal of avascularity caused by dead cortical sequestrae.

Utilizing the vitality and displacement of the fragments in a delayed union, nonunion, or pseudarthrosis, the site, and if there is infection with drainage, the author has devised his own classification of acquired (not congenital) nonunions (Table 15–1) (22). Based on this classification and the causes of the nonunion, the selective use of operative or electrical treatment can be determined.

If there is no deformity or only a mild acceptable one and the nonunion has vital ends without a major gap or synovial pseudarthrosis, PEMF treatment may be utilized. This is, of course, provided the patient is willing to accept

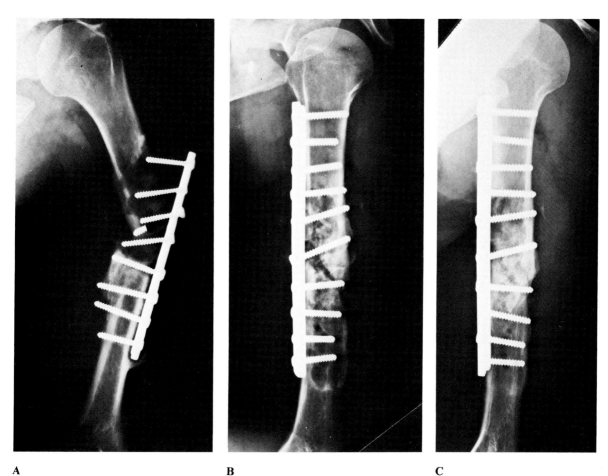

A   B   C

Figure 15-3 This 28-year-old male was in a motor vehicle accident in March 1980. He had an open fracture of the left humerus and was in a hanging cast for 10 weeks. In October 1980 he had a plate and bone bank graft. PEMF was applied from March to June 1981. The plate started to loosen in August 1981 (10 months after the operation). **A** June 1982. The patient had an oligotrophic pseudarthrosis, a loose plate and broken screw, motion, and a gap. **B** October 1982. He underwent removal of the old plate and screws, excision of the pseudarthrosis, excision of dead bone, opening of the medullary canals, insertion of an AO plate and lag screws, an iliac bone graft, and shingling. **C** May 1983. At 7 months after operation the nonunion has healed, and the patient has 90% motion of the shoulder and elbow.

attachment to an electrical outlet for 10–12 hr per day and the functional impairment that comes from long months of plaster immobilization. For those bones that are difficult to immobilize well with plaster, i.e., the humerus (Figure 15-4) or proximal third of the femur, PEMF electrical therapy becomes less attractive and the results are less reliable.

Treatment of PEMF Failures

Bassett et al. (4) recently reported the treatment of 45 failures of his PEMF electrical system to heal nonunions using bone grafts, further PEMF treatment, and plaster immobilization, with a 93% success rate. In the same article, he also reported on a series of nonunions where PEMF would most likely fail,

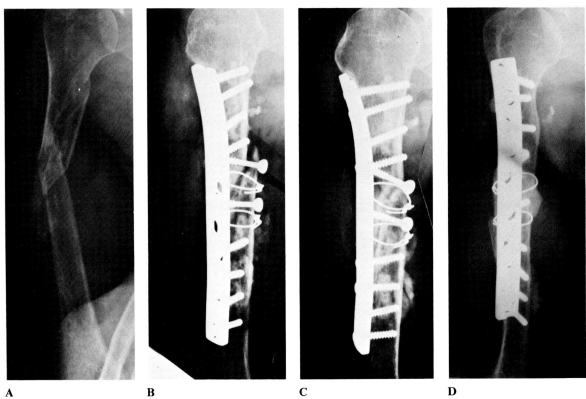

Figure 15-4 This 69-year-old female tripped and fell in October 1981, sustaining a fracture of the midshaft of the humerus. A hanging cast and velpeau were in position until October 1982. PEMF was applied from June to October 1982. **A** October 1982. At 1 year there was an atrophic nonunion, free motion, a gap, and malpositioning, with severe osteoporosis. **B** December 1982. Two months after surgery to insert an AO plate, lag screws, cerclage wires, an iliac bone graft, and cement in the screw holes to gain purchase in the porotic bone. The patient wore a sling and underwent active exercises. **C,D** AP and lateral x-rays 6 months later. The fracture has healed, and there is 75% function of the shoulder and 90% function of the elbow.

i.e., 38 patients with wide gaps, synovial pseudarthrosis, and/or malalignment. Again the treatment was bone grafting, cast immobilization, and PEMF treatment, with a success rate of 87%.

These are impressive results utilizing corticocancellous grafts—or pure cancellous bone when infection was present. No additional internal or external skeletal fixation was used, although some patients had metal devices still in place from prior unsuccessful procedures. Several loose or broken metal devices were removed at the time of bone grafting. In most patients, however, the primary immobilization was an appropriate plaster cast without weight-bearing for 2–12 months. Most of the nonunions in these two series were tibial and femoral (84%), and the median time to union in both groups was 4 months; 86% of the 14 fractures with infection united by this method.

Nothing specific, however, was mentioned in these two series (4) as to whether deformities were corrected or lengthened, how (except for plaster immobilization) these deformities were kept from recurring, or indeed what the rate of malunion actually was. To further address this point, two of the three cases that were presented to demonstrate healing of fractures by bone graft, PEMF, and cast immobilization showed persistent marked deformity by x-ray. In the third case—an infected nonunion of the humerus treated with a compression plate, bone graft, and PEMF—the alignment was good. This case was not included in the series described in the article, however, but was used only to demonstrate the "features of incorporation of the graft." Eight patients who were treated with PEMF initially and had refractures because of reduced cortical diameter were included in this series because "PEMF does not cause an increase in cortical diameter." Therefore, according to Bassett et al., if there is a major stress-concentrating defect, it should be bone-grafted and PEMF used to ensure early union and better cortical thickness.

Results of Operative Treatment

The author has seen 32 cases where PEMF has failed to heal a variety of nonunions. Of these, 17 have had operative treatment, the results of which are summarized in Table 15-2. Twelve of 14 have healed primarily (85.7%), two after a second operation. Two others have been operated on but are too recent to evaluate, although both patients are both doing well and healing is expected. One final nonunion, operated on 43 months ago, has slowly united, but in addition to operative plating, and bone graft, this patient also had PEMF for 9 months postoperatively and therefore really cannot be included in this purely operative series. There have been only two failures in the series—those two cases noted above that took two operative procedures to gain final union (14.3%). One of them was an infected nonunion of the tibia which had not united for 60 months, although the patient had 16 months of PEMF and seven previous operative procedures. The tibia did eventually unite with a plating of the fibula, with fibula protibia screws, shingling, and a bone graft, but she developed a stress fracture 5 months later and thus is classified a failure. The fracture required a vascularized rib graft and cast to finally unite 5 months later. The second case, an infected draining atrophic pseudarthrosis of the femur for 16 months, had three failed operative procedures and 9 months of PEMF. It still failed to unite even after an AO plate and iliac bone graft, although it healed and is dry 9 months after placement of an intramedullary rod and another iliac graft.

Table 15-2 Results of 17 Cases[a] of Internal Fixation of Nonunions After Unsuccessful PEMF (1979–1983)

| Site | No. of cases | Average healing time (mo) | Fracture healed | | | Failed | In progress |
			Not included[b]	After 1 operation	After 2 operations		
Tibia	9	7.7	1	6	1	1	1
Femur	4	6.6		2	1	1	1
Humerus	3	6.0		3			
Radius	1	14.0		1			
Total	17	7.6	1	12 (85.7%)	2	2 (14.3%)	2[c]

[a] Of the 17 cases, 7 were infected (5 draining), 13 were atrophic, and 4 were hypertrophic or oligotrophic.
[b] Had postoperative PEMF.
[c] Both cases have since healed.

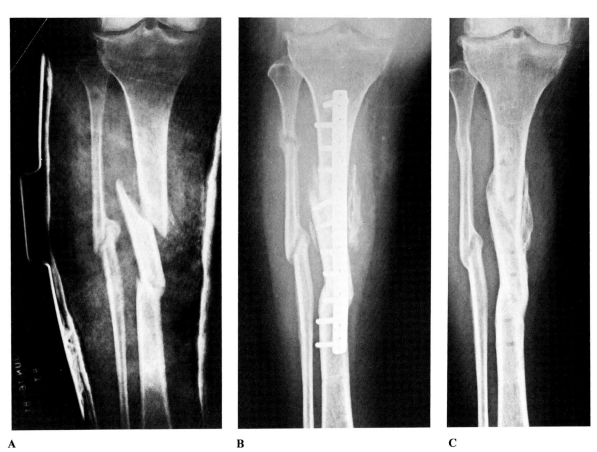

Figure 15–5 This 69-year-old female was struck by a car in September 1980. She was treated with pins, plaster, and a brace for 6 months. PEMF (EBI) was applied from March to August 1981. **A** June 1981. At 9 months after the fracture, there is still a segmental fracture (in plaster with PEMF) which has healed distally, but there is a relatively atrophic nonunion at the proximal fracture with overriding, 2-cm shortening, malpositioning, and free motion. **B** August 1981. At 11 months after the fracture. Note the postoperative AO plate, screws, and iliac bone graft with lengthening and realignment; no cast was used, and she healed 9 months later. **C** February 1983. At 5 months after the plate removal she had excellent function. Courtesy Dr. J. Rozbruch.

Operative Techniques to Achieve Union

The operative techniques used to achieve union in the above group of nonunions and pseudarthroses that failed to heal with PEMF stimulation included a variety of methods to obtain stable internal fixation and to stimulate bone repair. To give order to the multiplicity of treatments used in this series, the following regimens were followed:

1. *Hypertrophic vital nonunions* (elephant's foot callus) (Figure 15–2) require correction of any fixed deformity by osteotomy through the nonunion and then stable internal fixation. If the nonunion is movable, a tension band plate is applied to the convex side for correction of the deformity, or a tightly fitting IM rod is utilized after appropriate reaming. No additional bone graft is necessary because the callus already present is more than sufficient for union. Decortication or shingling should be used if callus is less abundant. No cast

or brace immobilization is needed if the patient is cooperative. Partial weight-bearing is allowed, but full weight-bearing is delayed until union is complete.

2. For *atrophic nonunions,* in addition to stable fixation with plates or IM rods, shingling or decortication (Figure 15–5) is necessary to reactivate the turned-off "bone-healing switch"; and a bone graft is inserted between the shingled osteoperiosteal fragments and the cortex. If a plate and screws are to be used in osteoporotic cortical bone, shingling will decrease the holding power of the screws. In these cases, shingling is kept to a thin shell of bone localized to 1–2 cm on either side of the fracture or is dispensed with entirely; petaling of the cortex adjacent to the plate is performed instead after plate application, and of course a bone graft added. When an IM rod is used in osteoporotic bone, care should be taken not to ream the inner cortex to such an extent that areas are left virtually devoid of cortex; and shingling is done cautiously.

For *atrophic pseudarthrosis* (Figure 15–6), if the deformity is to be corrected the medullary cavity should be opened with a drill or reamer to allow medullary mesenchymal cells to enter the fracture site. At the same time the pseudarthrosis tissue is either excised or compressed with the long compression device to achieve stable fixation.

Screws that do not hold in *severely osteoporotic cortical bone* (Figure 15–4) should be reinforced with liquid methylmethacrylate cement injected into the loose screw holes with a syringe. The screws are then replaced and tightened only after the cement has set. Care should be taken to prevent cement from entering the fracture by limiting the amount of cement injected into the screw holes, especially adjacent to the fracture, and curetting out any stray cement from between the fracture fragments or surrounding tissues. Instead, cancellous bone grafts are used liberally in and around the fracture gaps. If internal fixation is not adequate for stable fixation or if the patient is uncooperative, external plaster or a hinged brace support should be added after motion is regained.

For *metaphyseal–epiphyseal nonunions* (which we consider the most difficult), where (a) the small proximal or distal articular fragments are extremely porotic and often displaced, (b) the joint is stiff secondary to adhesions, muscle contracture, and malalignment, and (c) the pseudarthrosis is considered by nature to be the joint, the following formula has proved successful:

1. Perform a liberal arthrotomy to see the articular surface and realign the fragments, lyse adhesions, release periarticular contractures, remove loose bodies or fragments, frequently leave the capsule open, and gently manipulate the joint until it moves freely through a good arc of motion.

2. Reconstruct the articular block with lag or position screws replacing preliminary K wires. When screws do not hold in porotic bone, one can use liquid cement injected into the holes in order to gain better purchase in the weak bone.

3. Attach the reconstructed articular block to the metaphysis or shaft with plates (e.g., straight, blade, T, L, spoon) under compression. Stable fixation must be obtained or union will fail to occur. Bone grafts are rarely necessary unless gaps are present.

4. Start early active motion after preliminary splinting (depending on the amount of ligamentous repair or release) or immediately with a continuous passive motion machine. Weight-bearing is allowed late, with braces or hinged cast braces, when the fracture is uniting.

Synovial pseudarthrosis—diagnosed on x-rays, clinical motion at the fracture, and a cold cleft on the bone scan—may be compressed and stabilized with a plate and screws (Figure 15–1) or IM rod after reaming. It is best to excise the pseudarthrosis tissue, open the medullary canals, and then reduce

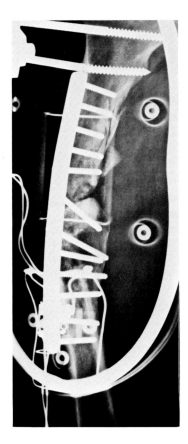

Figure 15-6 This 23-year-old male had a motor vehicle accident with subtrochanteric fracture of the right femur in December 1974 that healed with malunion and became infected. In April 1981 he underwent a multiplanar osteotomy with 5-cm lengthening with a Wagner apparatus and a lateral AO plate. No drainage occurred. In October 1982 the Wagner apparatus was removed. PEMF was applied from March 1982 to January 1983. **A** March 1982. PEMF (EBI) is present. Note the atrophic nonunion with the plate, Wagner apparatus, and Schanz pins in situ. **B** October 1982. There is no effect on the nonunion after 7 months of PEMF. **C** March 1983, 2 months after removal of the AO plate, excision of the fibrous nonunion, medullary reaming, insertion of an IM rod, AO plate, and screws, and iliac bone graft and shingling. **D,E** AP and lateral views in May 1983 (5 months postoperatively). Note the healing of the nonunion with bridging of the bone graft. The patient has 90% motion of the knee and is walking well.

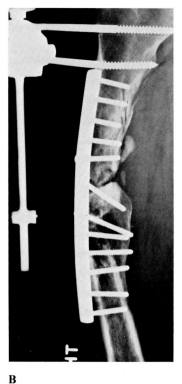

B

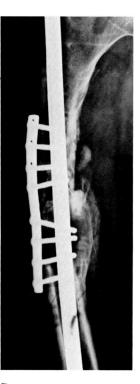

C

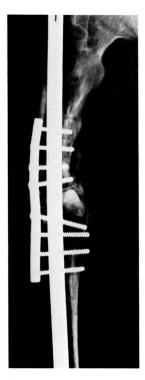

D

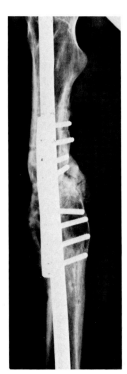

E

Internal Fixation of Nonunions After Unsuccessful Electromagnetic Stimulation

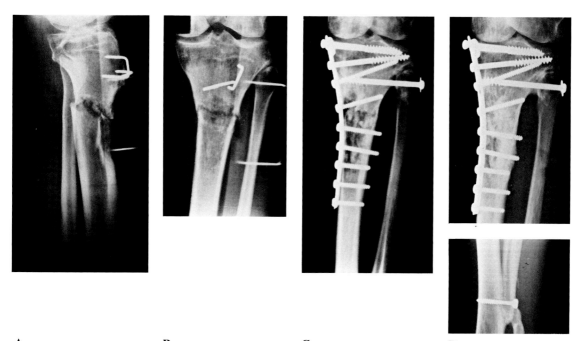

A   **B**   **C**   **D**

Figure 15-7 This 55-year-old male had radical resection of a malignant fibrous histiocytoma in June 1979 followed by 6500 rads of radiation. In December 1979 when playing tennis he jumped and sustained a fracture through the pathological bone. A cast and brace were applied. In November 1980 he showed a cold center on a bone scan. PEMF was applied December 1980 to October 1981 with a long cast and no weight-bearing. **A,B** Lateral and AP views in August 1981, after 8 months of PEMF. He was in a cast with an EBI marker. There was no change in the atrophic nonunion. Note the old staples in situ. **C** November 1981, 1 month after excision of necrotic bone, a fibula protibia synostosis with lag screw fixation proximal and distally, an iliac bone graft to fill the defect, and a AO buttress T plate. The fracture was healed by December 1982, 14 months after the operation. **D** June 1983. Note the solid union of the fracture and of the proximal and distal fibula protibia synostosis **(inset).** The patient is now walking well with 95% knee motion.

the fracture and internally fix as above. Shingling and bone grafts are indicated in the atrophic types or where a gap has to be filled.

Infected nondraining nonunions are treated like noninfected nonunions, but they should be debrided of any potentially infected fibrous or granulation tissue and shingled and bone-grafted if avascular bone is present (Figure 15.6). Sequestra, rarely present, are excised. Fixation is with neutralization plates and lag screws or by IM rods with reaming.

Infected draining nonunions are difficult. In the past the treatment was directed toward eradicating the infection first. This is done now only if the sepsis is caused by active abscess formation, in which case incision and drainage, debridement, and sequestrectomy with open packing or closed suction irrigation are performed to convert the active infection to a quiescent one. Attention is then directed toward healing the nonunion. This is done in the tibia by a bypass fibula protibia operation through a lateral approach at the level of the fracture several weeks later or by a proximal and distal tibiofibular synostosis procedure using screw fixation—and pure cancellous bone grafts (Figures 15–1 and 15–7). External unilateral frames with Schanz or threaded Steinman pins help stabilize the nonunion. Adjacent joint motion is encouraged during the healing period.

In the femur the bypass procedure is performed by shingling, liberal posterior-medial cancellous grafting, and stabilization by external fixators or a Wagner device (Figure 15–6).

After successful bypass bridging, the infection is eradicated by saucerization, sequestrectomy, radical excision of infected sinuses, fibrous and granulation tissue, and another cancellous bone graft. Closed suction irrigation is employed, or the wound is left open and packed until soft tissue healing occurs. External fixators are left in situ until bony continuity is strong enough to support weight-bearing with braces or cast braces. Joint motion and exercise are encouraged throughout the course of therapy.

Occasionally the bypass grafting and eradication of infection are done simultaneously (Figure 15–1). When large gaps are present or shortening demands lengthening prior to the above procedures, a vascularized fibula, iliac, or rib graft may be inserted by microvascular anastomosis. Supplemental iliac cancellous bone grafts and external fixators are usually necessary until the living bone graft matures and hypertrophies. If the former procedure is not available or not possible because of a lack of good arterial supply, iliac grafts may be used as a substitute to bridge large gaps. Appropriate antibiotics are used during the pre-, intra-, and postoperative periods to prevent recurrence or spread of infection but are not continued for long periods.

In all of the above procedures where malposition, angulation, malrotation, translocation, or combinations of these were present, care was taken to correct the deformity (Figures 15–1, 15–3, 15–5). Unacceptable major shortening was corrected by preliminary lengthening with the Wagner apparatus before definitive fixation was employed. Lengthening of lesser degrees was done as one procedure with the Müller distractor (Figure 15–5), the Wagner apparatus, or external fixator rods in a bilateral frame configuration at the time of internal fixation. Whichever procedure was used, however, it was mandatory to achieve a final mechanically neutral position of the limb rather than accept malpositioning or shortening.

Operative Armamentarium

The following modalities are available in the operative armamentarium for treating nonunions after failed PEMF stimulation:

Plates and screws: give stability against rotation (torsion), shear, and bending. Always use lag screws (interfragmentary compression) (Figure 15.2) and neutralization or tension band plates. Plates should be long and strong enough for sufficient stability.

IM rods: widest rod with reaming gives good stability against bending and shear but is poor against torsion. Therefore one frequently must use additional lag screws or plates for torsional stability (Figure 15.6).

External fixators (Wagner, AO, Hoffman, etc.): act as a *buttress* to bridge a gap or maintain length, a form of *neutralization* with lag screws across oblique or butterfly fractures, or a *tension band* with compression of transverse fractures. Pins should be of sufficient strength and number. No weight-bearing until callus ossification occurs; then partial weight-bearing with pins in situ, with compression added.

Bone grafts: essential for bypass bridging to stimulate osteogenesis, fill gaps, reinforce "medial" buttress (Figure 15.6), or obliterate dead space in infected cases. Vascularized grafts may be used for bridging large gaps.

Shingling and/or petaling: used to stimulate osteogenesis with grafts and start up the dormant process of bone healing (Figure 15–5).

Fibula protibia and bypass bridging: important tool for stabilizing tibial gaps or infected nonunions.

Cement: used in screw holes to gain better fixation in severely osteoporotic bone; never used in or around fracture ends (Figure 15–4).

Combinations of the above.

The operative treatment of patients with nonunions and pseudarthroses that fail to unite with electromagnetic stimulation (PEMF) has proved successful using the above modalities and techniques in 85% of the 17 cases in this series (Table 15–2). This confirms that union can be achieved in a high percentage of cases with the operative regimen described in this report even in patients with a deformity, motion, a gap, avascularity, synovial pseudarthrosis, or metaphyseal porotic bone.

REFERENCES

1. Anderson LD, Boyd HB, Johnston DS (1965). Changing concepts in the treatment of non union. Clin Orthop 43:37–54.
2. Bassett CAL, Chokshi HR, Hernandez E (1979). In: Electrical Properties of Bone and Cartilage, Experimental Effect and Clinical Applications. Grune & Stratton, New York.
3. Bassett CAL, Mitchell SN, Gaston SR (1981). Treatment of ununited tibial diaphyseal fractures with pulsing electromagnetic fields. J Bone Joint Surg 63A:511–523.
4. Bassett CAL, Mitchell SN, Schink MN (1982). Treatment of therapeutically resistant non unions with bone grafts and pulsing electromagnetic fields. J Bone Joint Surg 64A:1214–1220.
5. Bassett CAL, Pawluk RJ, Pilla AA (1974). Acceleration of fracture repair by electromagnetic fields: a surgically non-invasive method. Ann NY Acad sci 238:242–262.
6. Bassett CAL, Sharon MN, Gaston SR (1982). Pulsing electromagnetic field treatment in ununited fractures and failed arthrodeses. JAMA 247:623–628.
7. Brighton CT, Black J, Friedenberg ZB, et al. (1981). A multicenter study of the treatment of non-union with constant direct current. J Bone Joint Surg 63A:2–13.
8. Brighton CT, Friedenberg ZB, Zemsky LM, Pollis PA (1975). Direct-current stimulation of non union and congenital pseudarthrosis: exploration of its clinical application. J Bone Joint Surg 57A:368–377.
9. Connolly JF (1981). Selection, evaluation and indications for electrical stimulation of ununited fractures. Clin Orthop 161:39–53.
10. Esterhai JL, Brighton CT, Heppenstall RB, et al. (1981). Detection of synovial pseudarthrosis by ^{99m}Tc scintigraphy etc. Clin Orthop 161:15–23.
11. Fukuda E, Yasuda I (1957). On the piezoeffect of bone. J Physiol Soc Jpn 12:1158.
12. Jorgensen TE (1981). Asymmetrical slow-pulsating direct current. Clin Orthop 161:67–70.
13. Lechner F, Ascherl R, Uraus W (1981). Treatment of pseudarthroses with electrodynamic potentials of low frequency range. Clin Orthop 161:71–81.
14. Lente FD (1850). Cases of ununited fractures treated by electricity. NY J Med 5:317.
15. Mott V (1820). Two cases of ununited fractures successfully treated by stimulation. Med Surg Register 1 (Part 2):375.
16. Müller J, Schenk RK, Willinegger H (1968). Experimentelle Untersuchengen über die entstehung reaktiver Pseudoarthrosen am Hunderadius. Helv. Chir. Acta 35:301.
17. Müller ME (1965). Treatment of non unions by compression. Clin Orthop 43:83–92.
18. Paterson DC, Lewis GN, Cass CA (1980). Treatment of delayed union and nonunion with an implanted direct current stimulator. Clin Orthop 148:117–128.

19. Peltier LF (1981). A brief historical note on the use of electricity in the treatment of fractures. Clin Orthop 161:4–7.
20. Puranen J, Punto L (1981). Osteomedulloangiography: a method of estimating the consolidation prognosis of tibia shaft fractures. Clin Orthop 161:8–14.
21. Rosen H (1979). Compression treatment of pseudarthroses. Clin Orthop 138:154–166.
22. Rosen H (1979). Operative treatment of non unions of long bone fractures. Journal of Continuing Education in Orthopedics 7:13–39.
23. Schenk RK (1978). Histology of fracture repair and non union. Bulletin of the Swiss Association for Study of Internal Fixation, Bern.
24. Weber BG, Brunner C (1981). The treatment of nonunions without electrical stimulation. Clin Orthop 161:24–32.
25. Weber BG, Cech O (1976). Pseudarthrosis. Huber, Bern.
26. Yasuda I (1953). Piezoelectricity of living bone. J Kyoto Pref Univ Med 53:325.

Index

A

Acetabulum, femoral neck-shaft fractures and, 87

Angiography
  nonunion and, 196–97
  pelvic fractures and, 74–75

Ankle
  fibular fractures and, 145–51
  malleolar fracture of, 147–49

Anterior cord syndrome, 2, 11, 17

Antishock garment, pneumatic, 71–72

AO/ASIF screws
  knee dislocation repair and, 132
  triplane fractures of distal tibial epiphysis and, 169–70

AO external fixator, 35–55

Aorta, clamping of, 73

Aortogram, pelvic, 74

Arteriography
  internal iliac, 74
  knee dislocation and, 129

Arthrotomy, nonunion and, 203

ASIF external fixator, 35–55

Athlete, knee dislocation in, 125–34

Axis of limb, preoperative planning and, 100, 105, 111, 112

B

Bending axis, neutral, 58, 59

Bending moment, Ender nail and, 78

Brace
  knee, 129, 131, 132–33
  Somi, 15

Brown-Sequard syndrome, 3, 12, 15, 16

Burst fracture, cervical spine, 7, 11

Bypass bridging, nonunion and, 205–6, 207

C

Calcaneocuboid joint, 183
  plate for, 185

Calcaneus fractures, 173–92
  classification, 174–79
  comminuted, 178, 181
  complex, 176, 177, 184–86, 188
  impaction force and, 175–76
  internal fixation of, 173, 179–92
  mobility of subtalar joint and, 191–92
  poles of bone and, 176, 178
  radiographs of, 174, 176–82, 184, 186–90, 192
  results of treatment of, 190–91
  separation line of, 174
  surgical technique, 179–90
  three-fragment, 175
  tomograms of, 181, 182
  tongue type, 175, 176, 179
  two-fragment, 178–79, 182, 184

Calcification, electrical stimulation and, 194

Callus, 196
  classification of, 198
  controlled dynamic motion and, 143
  elephant's foot, 198, 202

Campbell exposure of humerus, 23, 24

Capitellum, 21, 27

209

Carpometatarsal joint fracture-dislocation,
52
Cartilage, electrical stimulation and, 194
Cassebaum exposure of humerus, 24, 25
repair of, 28
Casts
electrical stimulation and, 194, 195, 199–
201
femoral neck-shaft fractures and, 92, 93
humeral fractures and, 21, 33
knee dislocation and, 129, 131, 132–33
knee ligament injury and, 120
nonunion and, 199–201
spica, 72–73, 92
triplane fractures of distal tibial epiphysis
and, 167, 168
Cement, screws and, 203
Central cord syndrome, 2
Cephazolin, 147
Cervical spine, 1–18
burst fracture, 7, 11
classification of syndromes associated
with injury of, 1–2
compression fracture, 2, 7
decision-making and stabilization
method, 8–12
mid and lower cervical spine, 10–12
upper cervical spine, 8–10
decompression urgency and, 17–18
diagnostic aids, 12–13
disc protrusion, 13, 16
facet injuries, 7, 11
Gardner-Wells tongs and, 13, 17
halo and halo vest for, 15
initial treatment of, 8
lateral mass fracture, 7, 12
myelography and, 12–13, 15–17
neurological evaluation, 1–3
odontoid fractures, 4, 9–10
pars interarticularis C2 fracture, 4, 10
patterns of fracture of, 3–8
mid and lower, 7
upper, 3–4
Philadelphia collar and, 15
posterior ligamentous disruption, 2, 7,
11–12
ring fracture, 4, 8–9
Somi brace, 15
teardrop fracture, 7, 11
technical considerations, 13–17
tomography, 12
wiring of neural arches, 9–10
Clamps
aortic, 73
wrist, 38
Coagulopathy, pelvic fractures and, 70
Collateral ligaments, knee, 132
Colles fracture, 43
Comminuted fractures
calcaneus, 178, 181
femoral, 94–95
hand, 65
humeral, 21, 27, 29, 34

tibial, 136, 140–41
wrist, 35–36
Compression fracture, cervical spine, 2, 7
Compression plates
electrical stimulation and, 194
femoral neck-shaft fractures and, 88, 89,
94–96
humeral supracondylar fracture and, 25
nonunion and, 195, 203
Computerized tomography
cervical injury and, 13
triplane fractures of tibia and, 158–59,
165
Controlled dynamic motion, 143
Cooperman triplane fracture, 154, 161
Corrective surgery of posttraumatic deformities, preoperative planning for,
99–116
compound deformity and, 108–14
discussion on, 115
materials, 100–101
methods, 101–3
results, 115
simple deformity and, 103–8
Corticospinal tracts, 2, 3
Crash protocol, pelvic fractures and, 73–
74
Cruciate ligaments, 131–32
Crush injuries
fibular, 146
forearm, 48

D
Dashboard injury, 86, 87
DC plate, humeral, 23, 25, 27
Decompression, cervical cord injury and,
17–18
Deformities, posttraumatic, preoperative
planning for correction of, 99–116
Disc protrusion, cervical, 13, 16
Dislocation, knee, 125–34
Distraction, wrist, 35–55
Drawings, preoperative, 100–107, 111–13
Drilling
femoral Ender nailing and, 80
hand tension bands and, 63
olecranon osteotomy repair and, 28
tibial shaft fractures and, flexible intra-
medullary nailing of, 137
wrist wiring and, 37
Dynamic motion, controlled, 143
Dystrophy, Sudeck's, 54

E
Edema, spinal cord, 2
Effusion, knee, 119, 121
Electrical stimulation, 193–95, 199–201
failure of, treatment of, 199–201
knee repair and, 132, 133
methods of, 193–94
problems with, 195

Index   **211**

Electrical stimulation *(cont.)*
  results of, 194–95
  theoretical concepts, 194
Elephant's foot callus, 198, 202
Embolization, pelvic fractures and, 74–75
Ender nailing
  of femoral shaft fractures, 93, 95
  of intertrochanteric fractures, 77–83, 95
    complications, 81–83
    external rotation deformity and, 81
    hip joint penetration and, 82
    pin prominence at knee and, 82
    rationale for, 79
    supracondylar fracture and, 82
    technique, 79–81
Epicondylar ridges, humeral, 21
Exercises, knee, 132–33
External fixation
  fibular fracture, 145–51
  pelvic fracture, 72
  wrist fracture, 35–55
External fixators, nonunion and, 206
External rotation
  Tillaux fracture and, 165
  triplane fractures and, 163–64

F
Facet injuries, cervical, 7, 11
Femur, 77–123
  axis of, 100, 111, 112
  comminuted fractures of, 94–95
  compression plates for, 88, 89, 94–96
  dashboard injury to, 86, 87
  Ender nailing of, 77–83, 93, 95
    complications, 81–83
    external rotation deformity and, 81
    hip joint penetration and, 82
    pin prominence at knee and, 82
    rationale for, 79
    supracondylar fracture and, 82
    technique, 79–81
  graft for, 89, 90, 94–96
  hip fracture concomitant with fracture
    of, 85–96
    classification and preferred treatment,
      93–96
    experience with, 90–91
    historical review, 85–87
    management, 87–90
    neck fracture and stable shaft fracture,
      93–94
    neck fracture and unstable shaft frac-
      ture, 94–95
    pathomechanics, 87
    results of treatment of, 91–93
    stable pertrochanteric fracture and
      stable shaft fracture, 95
    stable pertrochanteric fracture and
      unstable shaft fracture, 95
    unstable pertrochanteric fracture and
      stable shaft fracture, 95

    unstable pertrochanteric fracture and
      unstable shaft fracture, 96
  intertrochanteric fractures, 77–83
  knee injuries and, 86, 87, 117–23
    diagnosis, 118–20
    material, 117–18
    treatment options, 120–21
  malunion of, 204
  nonunion of, 204, 206
    neck fracture and, 91, 92
  osteotomy of, 78, 95
    planning of, 105, 107, 113
  preoperative planning of corrective sur-
    gery for posttraumatic deformities
    of, 99–116
    compound deformity and, 108–14
    discussion on, 115
    materials, 100–101
    methods, 101–3
    results, 115
    simple deformity and, 103–8
  radiographs of, 102, 103, 109, 113
    knee ligament injury and, 119, 120,
      122
    neck-shaft fractures and, 88–92
  rotational malalignment of, 108–14
  stabilizing pins for, diagnostic, 119–20
  stress testing and, 119
  tracings of, 104–7, 111–13
  traction for, 92, 93, 120–22
  valgus deformity and, 103–8
Fibrocartilage, electrical stimulation and,
  194
Fibula, 145–51
  biomechanics, 145, 146
  external fixation of, 145–51
    case reports, 147–50
    conclusions on, 151
    method, 146–47
  protibia operation, 205, 207
  radiographs of, 148–50
  screws in, 146
    triplane fracture and, 169
  supination-eversion injuries and, 163,
    164
  syndesmosis injury and, 147, 148
  tibial fracture nailing and, 138
  triplane fractures of distal tibial epiphysis
    and, 154–57, 161, 167–69
Figure-of-eight bands, 59
Flexible nailing, tibial shaft, 135–44
Foot, fracture-dislocation of, 52
Frame fixation of wrist, 38–39
  without crossing joint, 41, 44–45

G
Gardner-Wells tongs, 13, 17
Gel foam, pelvic bleeding and, 74
Genicular arteries, 126
Geniculate artery, medial, 80
Goniometer, 101
Grafts
  cervical teardrop/burst fractures and, 11
  femoral, 89, 90, 94–96
  for nonunion, 199–201, 203, 205, 206

Grafts (cont.)
  odontoid process, 10
  preoperative planning for, 107
  saphenous vein, knee dislocation and,
    129
  tibial, 53
  ulnar, 50
Grosse-Kempf nail, 95
Growth plate, triplane fractures of distal
    tibial epiphysis and, 162
Gunshot wounds, humeral fractures and,
    29, 31

H
Halo, 15
Halo vest, 15
  odontoid fracture and, 9
Hamstrings, knee dislocations and, 133
Hand, tension bands for, 57–67
  background of, 57–58
  complex fractures, 65
  long spiral oblique fractures, 64–65
    metacarpal, 64
    phalangeal, 64–65
  principle of, 58–61
  short spiral oblique fractures, 65
  summary of, 66
  techniques for, 61–63
  transversely oriented fractures, 63–
    64
    metacarpal, 63
    phalangeal, 63–64
Hangman's fracture, 4, 10
Head-holding device, 15
Hematoma, humeral fractures and, 23
Hemorrhage
  knee, 126
  pelvic fractures and, 70–75
  spinal cord, 2
Hip fractures. See also Pelvic fractures.
  Ender pins and. See Ender nailing.
  ipsilateral femoral shaft fractures and.
    See Femur, hip fracture concomi-
    tant with fracture of.
Hoffmann pins, 146, 148
Holt nail, 77
Humerus, 21–34
  Campbell exposure of, 23, 24
  Cassebaum exposure of, 24, 25
  comminuted fractures of, 21, 27, 29, 34
  complications of fractures of, 33
  DC plate and, 23, 25, 27
  discussion on, 33–34
  internal fixation of fractures of, 24–28
    intercondylar, 27–28
    supracondylar, 24–27
  nonunion of, 32, 33, 199, 200
  olecranon osteotomy and, 24, 25
    repair of, 28
  operative technique for, 22–23
  radial distraction and, 42
  radial nerve palsy and, 29, 31, 33

  radiographs of, 22, 23, 25–28, 30–32
  results of repair of, 28–32
  supracondylar and intercondylar frac-
    tures of, 21–34

I
Iliac arteries, bleeding from, 74
Iliac arteriography, internal, 74
Iliotibial band, knee reconstruction and,
    132
Image intensifier
  Ender nailing and, 79, 80
  flexible intramedullary nailing of tibial
    shaft fractures and, 136, 137
IM rods, 202, 203, 206
Incisions
  calcaneus fractures and, 183
  Ender nailing of femur and, 80
  hand tension bands and, 63
  humeral repair, 22–23
  intramedullary nailing of tibial shaft
    fractures and, 137
Infection
  calcaneus fractures and, 190
  forearm, 47, 50
  humeral fractures and, 32, 33
  nonunion and, 195, 198, 205–6
  tibial shaft nailing and, 143, 144
Instron testing machine, 59
Intercondylar fractures of humerus, 21–
    34
Intercondylar notch, knee dislocation re-
    pair and, 130, 131
Internal fixation
  calcaneus fracture, 173, 179–92
  femoral, Ender nailing for, 77–83
  femoral neck-shaft fracture, 86–96
  hand fracture, 57–67
  humeral fracture, 24–28
    intercondylar, 27–28
    supracondylar, 24–27
  of nonunions, 195, 201–7
  pelvic fracture, 73
  strain recording of, 59
  triplane fractures of distal tibial epiphysis
    and, 168–69
Interosseous ligament, calcaneus fractures
    and, 174–75
Interphalangeal joints, tension bands and,
    62
Intertrochanteric fractures, Ender nailing
    of, 77–83, 95
Intervertebral disc protrusion, cervical, 13,
    16
Intramedullary nailing, flexible, for tibial
    shaft fractures, 135–44
Intraosseous venography, 196, 197

J
Jefferson fracture, 4, 8–9
Jones bandage, 81

Index **213**

K

Kirschner wires
  corrective surgery for deformities and, 103, 112–13
  humeral fractures and, 27
  tension bands for hand and, 59, 63–67
  wrist fractures and, 36–41
Knee
  axis of, 100, 105
  cast brace for, 129, 131, 132–33
  dashboard injury, 86, 87
  dislocation of, 125–34
    in athlete, 125–34
    classification, 126
    complications, 128–29
    diagnosis, 126–28
    summary, 133–34
    surgical anatomy, 126
    treatment, 129–33
  effusion of, 119, 121
  Ender pin prominence at, 82
  exercises for, 132–33
  hyperextension injury, 126
  iliotibial band in repair of, 132
  ipsilateral hip-femoral shaft fractures and, 86, 87
  ligament injuries, 117–23
    dislocations and, 126, 130–32
    femoral fractures and, 117–23
  meniscus, 126, 131
  nerve injury and, 126, 128, 129
  passive motion and, 132, 133
  radiographs of
    dislocation and, 127
    ligament injury and, 119, 120, 122
  stress testing, 119, 122
  traction and, 120–22, 129
  vascular structures of, 126, 128, 129, 131
Knowles pins
  femoral neck-shaft fractures and, 85, 91–94
  nonunion and, 92
Kuntscher nail, 78, 79

L

Lachman's test, 119
Lag screws
  calcaneus fractures and, 185
  humeral supracondylar fracture and, 25–27
  nonunion and, 203, 206
  olecranon osteotomy repair and, 28
Lambotte's hook, 184
Lateral cord syndrome, 3
Ligamentotaxis, 35
Ligaments
  cervical spine, 2, 7, 11–12
  knee, 126, 130–32
    femoral fractures and, 117–23
Looped bands, 59, 63

M

Malleolus, medial, fracture of, 147–49
  triplane fractures and, 154–57
Malunion
  electrical stimulation and, 195
  femoral, 204
  tibial shaft nailing and, 144
Marmor triplane fracture, 153–56, 160–61
Median nerve, wrist fractures and, 53
Mediview viewbox, 101
Meniscus, 126, 131
Metacarpals
  fixation of, 36–39
    triangular, 41, 46–47
  osteotomy of, tension bands and, 59
  tension bands and, 63–65
    complex fractures and, 65
    long spiral oblique fractures and, 64
    short spiral oblique fractures and, 65
    transverse fractures and, 63
Metacarpophalangeal joints, tension bands and, 62
Metaphyseal-epiphyseal nonunion, 195, 203
Mineralization, electrical stimulation and, 194
Minilaparotomy, 71
Monroe tracing paper, 101
Müller distractor, 206
Myelography, cervical spine injury and, 12–13, 15–17

N

Nails
  Ender
    femoral shaft fractures and, 93, 95
    intertrochanteric fractures and, 77–83, 95
    femoral neck-shaft fractures and, 90, 91, 93
    flexible intramedullary, for tibial shaft fractures, 135–44
    Grosse-Kempf, 95
    Holt, 77
    Rush dictum for, 140
    Sarmiento, 77
Nerve roots, 3, 11
  C8, 2
Neural arches, cervical, wiring of, 9–10
Neurological evaluation
  cervical spine injuries and, 1–3
  knee dislocation and, 128
Neutral bending axis, 58, 59
Nonunion, 193–207
  atrophic, 195, 203
  classification, 196, 197–99
  diagnostic tools used for, 196–97
  electrical stimulation for, 193–95
  femoral, 91, 92, 204, 206
  grafts for, 199–201, 203, 205, 206
  humeral fracture, 32, 33, 199, 200
  hypertrophic, 202–3
  infection and, 195, 198, 205–6

Nonunion *(cont.)*
  metaphyseal-epiphyseal, 195, 203
  oligotrophic, 198, 199
  operative treatment of, 202–7
    armamentarium for, 206–7
    rationale for, 196
    results of, 195, 201
    techniques, 202–6
  osteoporosis and, 203
  plaster immobilization for, 199–201
  radiographs of, 198–200, 202, 204, 205
  tibial, 143, 201, 205
  wrist fracture, 54

O

Odontoid fractures, 4, 9–10
Olecranon osteotomy, 24, 25
  repair of, 28
Os calcis. *See also* Calcaneus fractures.
  pin fixation of, 52
Osteitis, forearm, 47, 50
Osteomedulloangiography, 196
Osteomyelitis, tibial shaft nailing and, 143, 144
Osteoporosis
  Ender nailing of femoral fracture and, 79, 82
  nonunion and, 203
Osteotomy
  femoral, 78, 95
    planning of, 105, 107, 113
  metacarpal, tension bands and, 59
  nonunions and, 202
  olecranon, 24, 25
    repair of, 28
  preoperative planning of, 102, 105, 107, 113

P

Palsy, radial nerve, 29, 31, 33
Paper for preoperative drawings, 101
Pars interarticularis C2 fracture, 4, 10
Passive motion, knee dislocation repair and, 132, 133
Peiro's fracture, 156, 160, 161
Pelvic fractures, 69–75
  angiography, 74–75
  coagulopathy and, 70
  hemorrhage and, 70–75
  management, 71
  pneumatic antishock garment and, 71–72
  reduction of, 72–73
  review of cases, 70
  shock and, 70, 71–72
  surgical control of, 73–74
    crash protocol, 73–74
    major vessel injury, 73
    open fractures, 73
  tamponade and, 71
  unstable vs. stable, 69, 70

PEMF (pulsing electromagnetic fields), 194–95, 199–201
Perilunar fracture-dislocation, 41
Peroneal nerve, knee injury and, 126, 128, 129
Peroneal tendons, calcaneus fractures and, 183
Phalanges
  long spiral oblique fractures of, 64–65
  tension bands for, 63–65
  transverse fractures of, 58, 63–64
Philadelphia collar, 15
Pilon injuries, fibular, 145, 146
Pin fixation
  femoral, 90–94
    Ender method of, 78–83
    nonunion and, 92
  fibular fracture, 146–51
  os calcis, 52
  tension bands for hand and, 63–67
  tibial, 53
Planning, preoperative, of corrective surgery, 99–116
Plantar flexion, triplane fractures and, 163–64
Plates
  compression. *See* Compression plates.
  DC, humeral fracture and, 23, 25, 27
  electrical stimulation and, 194
  femoral, 78, 88, 89, 94–96
  nonunion and, 195, 203, 206
  tubular, humeral fracture and, 26, 27
  ulnar, 47, 48, 50
  Y vitallium, calcaneus fracture and, 185
Pneumatic antishock garment, 71–72
Popliteal artery, 126
  exploration of, 128
Popliteal tendon, 132
Posterior cord syndrome, 3
Posterolateral corner of knee, 132
Preoperative planning of corrective surgery for posttraumatic deformities, 99–116
  compound deformity and, 108–14
  discussion on, 115
  materials, 100–101
  methods, 101–3
  results, 115
  simple deformity and, 103–8
Protek templates, 102
Pseudarthrosis, 196, 198
  atrophic, 203
  oligotrophic, 199
  operative treatment of, 195
  radiographs of, 196, 199
  synovial, 196, 203–5
Pulsing electromagnetic fields (PEMF), 194–95, 199–201

Q

Quadriceps, exercises for, knee dislocations and, 133

Index 215

R
Radial nerve palsy, 29, 31, 33
Radiography
  calcaneus fractures and, 174, 176–82,
      184, 186–90, 192
  cervical spine injuries and, 2, 4–17
  femoral, 102, 103, 109, 113
    knee ligament injury and, 119, 120,
        122
    neck-shaft fractures and, 88–92
  fibular fracture and, 148–50
  hand fractures and, 62, 66
  humeral fractures and, 22, 23, 25–28, 30–
      32
  knee, 119, 120, 122
    dislocation and, 127
  nonunions and, 198–200, 202, 204, 205
  preoperative planning and, 100, 102, 103,
      109, 113
  pseudarthrosis and, 196, 199
  tibial shaft nailing and, 138–41
  tibial triplane fracture and, 154, 166–69
  tracings of, 100–107, 111–13
  wrist fracture and, 40, 42, 44, 46, 48
Radioisotope studies, pseudarthrosis and,
    196
Radius
  distal fractures of, 35. See also Wrist.
  fixation of, 36–39
    humerus-ulna fixation and, 42, 48
    to second metacarpal, 36–39
    to third metacarpal, 39
    triangular, to first and second metacar-
        pals, 41, 46–47
Richards plate, 90
Ring fracture, cervical spine, 4, 8–9
Rods
  IM, 202, 203, 206
  wrist, 38–41
Rush dictum, 140

S
Sacroiliac disruption. See Pelvic fractures.
Salter-Harris fractures, 153–57, 160, 163,
    164
Saphenous vein graft, knee dislocation and,
    129
Sarmiento nail, 77
Screws
  calcaneus, 184, 185
  cement to reinforce, 203
  femoral, 78, 88–90, 95–96
  fibular, 146, 169
  humeral supracondylar fracture and, 25–
      27
  knee dislocation repair and, 132
  malleolar, medial, 147, 148
  nonunion and, 203, 206
  osteoporosis and, 203
  preoperative planning and, 102–3
  sliding, femoral fractures and, 78
  triplane fractures of distal tibial epiphysis
      and, 169–70

Shingling, nonunion and, 203
Shock, pelvic fractures and, 70, 71–72
  pneumatic antishock garment and, 71–
      72
Sinus tarsi, 174
Skin necrosis, calcaneus fractures and, 190
Somi brace, 15
Spica cast, 72–73
  femoral neck-shaft fracture and, 92
Spinal cord
  anterior syndrome, 2, 11, 17
  central syndrome, 2
  decompression of, 17–18
  lateral (Brown-Sequard) syndrome, 3,
      12, 15, 16
  nerve root function, 3, 11
  posterior syndrome, 3
Spine, cervical. See Cervical spine.
Spinothalamic tract, 2, 3
Splints, hand tension bands and, 62
Steinman pin
  femoral stabilization and, 119
  nonunion and, 92
Strain recording model, 59, 60
Stress testing, knee ligament, 119, 122
Subtalar joint, 173–74
  exposure of, 183
  impaction of, 175
  internal fixation of, 183–85
  mobility of, 191–92
  separation line and, 174
Sudeck's dystrophy, 54
Supination-eversion injuries, triplane frac-
    tures and, 163–64
Synthes device, 90

T
Talus, calcaneus fractures and, 175
Tamponade, pelvic fractures and, 71
Teardrop fracture, cervical spine, 7, 11
Templates, preoperative planning and, 102
Tension bands, hand, 57–67
  complex fractures and, 65
  long spiral oblique fractures and, 64–65
  principles of, 58–61
  short spiral oblique fractures and, 65
  techniques for, 61–63
  transversely oriented fractures and, 63–
      64
Thalamus, 173
  impaction of, 175–76
  reconstruction of, 183–85
  separation line and, 174
Tibia
  axis of, 100
  comminuted fractures, 136, 140–41
  external fixation of, 53
  flexible intramedullary nails for, 135–
      44
    clinical experience with, 142–44
    complications, 142–43
    concluding remarks on, 143–44

Tibia (cont.)
    indications, pitfalls and errors, 139–42
    instruments for, 136
    operative technique, 136–39
    selection of nails, 138–39
    stable fractures and, 135–36
    unstable fractures and, 136
  graft of, 53
  knee dislocation and, 129
  nonunion of, 143, 201, 205
  oblique fractures, 135, 139, 140
  radiographs of, nailing and, 138–41
  sliding of fracture fragments of, 139–40
  spiral fracture, 138–40
  Tillaux fracture, 156, 163, 165–66
  traction for femoral fractures and, 120–22
  transverse fractures, 135, 139
  triplane fractures of distal epiphysis of, 153–70
    anatomy, 153–62
    Cooperman, 154, 161
    CT scans of, 158–59, 165
    definition of, 153
    diagnosis, 164–66
    growth plate maturation and, 162
    historical review, 153
    Marmor, 153–56, 160–61
    mechanism, 163–64
    medial, 160
    Peiro, 156, 160, 161
    prognosis, 170
    radiographs of, 154, 166–69
    Salter-Harris types, 153–57, 160, 163, 164
    summary, 170
    tomograms of, 154, 157, 165
    treatment, 167–70
Tibial nerve, knee injury and, 126, 128
Tibiofibular syndesmosis, fibular fractures and, 147, 148
Tibiotalar joint, biomechanics of, 145
Tillaux fracture, 156, 163, 165–66
Tomography
  calcaneus fracture and, 181, 182
  cervical spine, 12
  computed. See Computerized tomography.
  triplane fractures of distal tibial epiphysis and, 154, 157, 165
Tongs, Gardner-Wells, 13, 17
Tongue type fracture of calcaneus, 175, 176, 179
Tracing, x-ray, preoperative planning and, 100–107, 111–13
Traction
  cervical spine injuries and, 11, 13, 17
  femoral fractures and, 120–22
    of neck-shaft, 92, 93
  Gardner-Wells, 13, 17
  knee dislocation and, 129
  knee ligament injury and, 120–21

Transfusions, pelvic fractures and, 71
Triangular fixation of radius to first and second metacarpals, 41, 46–47
Triceps, humeral fractures and, 23, 24
Triplane fractures. See Tibia, triplane fractures of distal epiphysis of.
Trochanteric fractures, Ender nailing of, 77–83
Trochlea, humeral, 21, 27
Tubular plate, humeral fractures and, 26, 27

U
Ulna
  osteitis of, 50
  plate fixation of, 47, 48, 50
  radial distraction and, 42
Ulnar nerve, humeral fractures and, 23, 24

V
Valgus
  calcaneus reconstruction and, 184
  Ender nailing and, 80
  femoral osteotomy and, 78, 95
  nonunion and, 198
  preoperative planning for corrective surgery for, 103–8
  tibial shaft nailing and, 141, 144
Varus, stress view of knee in, 120, 122
Vastus medialis, Ender nailing and, 80
Venography, intraosseous, 196, 197
Viewbox, preoperative drawing and, 100–101

W
Wagner apparatus, 204, 206
Weber fractures, 146
Wires
  corrective surgery for deformities and, 103, 112–13
  humeral fractures and, 27
  neural arch, cervical, 9–10
  olecranon osteotomy repair and, 28
  tension band, hand fractures and, 58–67
  wrist fracture, 36–41
Wrist, 35–55
  aftercare of fractures of, 47, 50
  complications of fractures of, 50, 53–54
  distraction in any desired position, 40, 43–44
  external fixation of, 35–55
  frame fixation without crossing the joint, 41, 44–45
  humerus-radius-ulna internal fixation and, 42, 48
  instrumentation for, 36

Index

Wrist *(cont.)*
    neutral position of, fixation in, 36–
        40
    nonunion of, 54
    radiographs of, 40, 42, 44, 46, 48
    radius-second metacarpal fixation of, 36–
        39
    radius-third metacarpal fixation of,
        39
    results of treatment of, 55

surgical technique for, 36–42
triangular fixation of radius to first and
    second metacarpals, 41, 46–47

X
X-rays. *See* Radiography.

Y
Y-plate, calcaneus fracture and, 185

Techniques in Orthopaedics
Editorial Board

Lester Borden, M.D.
Head, Section of Adult Reconstructive Orthopaedic
Surgery
Cleveland Clinic
9500 Euclid Avenue
Cleveland, Ohio 44106

Kenneth E. DeHaven, M.D.
Professor of Orthopaedics
Head, Section of Athletic Medicine
University of Rochester Medical Center
601 Elmwood Avenue
Rochester, New York 14642

Lawrence D. Dorr, M.D.
Consultant, Arthritis Service
Rancho Los Amigos Hospital
7601 East Imperial Highway
Downey, California 90242;
Southwestern Orthopaedic Medical Group
501 East Hardy Street
Inglewood, California 90301

David S. Hungerford, M.D.
Associate Professor of Orthopaedic Surgery
Johns Hopkins Hospital

601 N. Broadway Street
Baltimore, Maryland 21239;
Chief, Division of Arthritis Surgery
Good Samaritan Hospital
5601 Loch Raven Blvd.
Baltimore, Maryland 21239

William Grana, M.D.
Director, Oklahoma Center for Athletes
711 Stanton L. Young Blvd.
Suite 310
Oklahoma City, Oklahoma 73104

Douglas W. Jackson, M.D.
Director, Southern California Center for Sports
Medicine
2760 Atlantic
Long Beach, California 90806

James Kellam, M.D.
Division of Orthopaedics
Sunnybrook Hospital
2075 Bayview Avenue
Toronto, Ontario M4N 3M5
Canada

John B. McGinty, M.D.
Clinical Professor of Orthopaedic Surgery
Tufts University School of Medicine
Boston, Massachusetts;
Chief, Orthopaedic Surgery
Newton-Wellesley Hospital
2000 Washington Street
Newton Lower Falls, Massachusetts 02162

Chitranjan S. Ranawat, M.D.
Professor of Orthopaedic Surgery
Hospital for Special Surgery
525 W. 70th Street
New York, New York 10021

David Seligson, M.D.
Kosair Professor and Chief
Division of Orthopaedics
University of Louisville School of Medicine
550 South Jackson Street
Louisville, Kentucky 40292

Phillip G. Spiegel, M.D.
Chairman and Professor
Department of Orthopaedic Surgery
University of South Florida
12901 N. 30th Street
Box 36
Tampa, Florida 33612

Richard B. Welch, M.D.
Senior Consultant
San Francisco Orthopaedics Training Program
4141 Geary Blvd.
San Francisco, California;
Chief, Arthritis Clinic
St. Mary's Hospital
San Francisco, California 94118

Robert A. Winquist, M.D.
Orthopaedic Physicians, Inc., P.S.
Suite 1600
901 Boren Avenue
Seattle, Washington 98104